Tired all the Time

Defeating Dysautonomia

A practical guide for patients and families
to managing POTS and related conditions

Dr Brendan B Hanrahan, MBBS FRACP

To my wife, my life, my sweetness

First Edition 2025

First Edition.

ISBN: 978-1-7637445-1-6

Self-Published.

http://aionhealth.com.au/dysautonomia-resources

Disclaimer: This guide is not intended as a substitute for the medical advice of physicians. Any action you take based on the content of this guide is strictly at your own risk. Readers should consult with a licensed medical professional before making any healthcare decisions or changes to their treatment plans. The author and publisher are not liable for any damages or adverse outcomes resulting from the use or misuse of the information presented. The reader should regularly consult a physician in matters relating to their health and particularly with respect to any symptoms that may require diagnosis or medical attention.

While the author has made every effort to provide accurate information at the time of publication, neither the publisher nor the author assumes any responsibility for errors, inaccuracies, omissions, or any inconsistency herein. Any slights of people, places, or organisations are unintentional.

Book Design by Brendan Hanrahan.
Cover Design by Brendan Hanrahan.

Contents

Tired all the Time
Defeating Dysautonomia

A practical guide for patients and families
to managing POTS and related conditions

It is also not meant to be a comprehensive exhaustive text on the conditions, their causes, or all the details of past, current and potential therapies — that would be a much, much longer volume. It is rather intended to focus on the essentials of assisting people new to the conditions to work out what's going on and hopefully help people rapidly find the best available clinical management(s) of common Dysautonomias.

1

It doesn't cover every possible situation, but is intended as a place to start and should provide sufficient guidance for the majority of cases.

This guide is intended primarily for patients and those who care for them, and may be shared with their treating team. The goal is to speed diagnosis and implementation of optimal therapy, by complementing the knowledge, experience and expertise their regular doctors already have.

<u>A style comment</u>: If I seem to be belabouring a point and repeating myself — it's deliberate. People with these conditions almost universally report experiencing "brain fog." In my clinical experience, I often repeat important points several timnaryes during an appointment and provide printed summary handouts, only to still receive calls days later seeking clarification of those same points. So while trying to make this guide as accessible as possible, I've intentionally included some moderate repetition to aid comprehension.

Similarly, I've tried to keep to "non-medical" language. However, at times it's necessary to use precise medical terminology rather than simpler alternatives. When this occurs, you'll find clear definitions in the glossary at the end of the guide.

<u>A Note on Accessibility</u>: Dysautonomia and Attention-Deficit/Hyperactivity Disorder (ADHD) occur more frequently in this guide's likely readership than in the general population, and many individuals with ADHD also experience dyslexia. If you find reading challenging, consider changing your e-reader settings to a dyslexia-friendly font. This simple adjustment can significantly improve readability and your overall reading experience.

Most e-readers offer font options designed to be more easily readable for people with dyslexia.

Common dyslexia-friendly fonts include OpenDyslexic, Dyslexie, and Comic Sans MS.

We're committed to making this important information as accessible as possible to all readers. If you have suggestions for improving the accessibility of this guide, please don't hesitate to reach out.

Introduction

You're tired all the time. You don't have the energy others your age seem to have, and when you do push through for a big day, you crash afterward — often for several days. You have brain fog, struggle with short-term memory, and find yourself searching for words. You may have other features like dizziness or fainting, awareness of your heart beating or racing, gastrointestinal troubles, feelings of pooling of blood and congestion in the legs or hands, colour changes in the hands and/or legs, abnormal sensations in your arms, head, the shoulders, or anywhere from the belly button up. Headaches are common and you struggle to sleep well. You may even have issues with temperature regulation. You feel lousy after a flight or a long car trip despite just sitting there. You carry a water bottle and a notebook wherever you go. If you do happen to get intravenous fluids for some reason you feel great for a few hours or a couple of days. With any combination of these and many more, it is quite possible you might have a Dysautonomia.

Dysautonomia is a Greek word for the Automatic Nervous Systems (ANS) of the body being detuned or "wonky". Doctors call this the Autonomic Nervous System[1], and these are the systems that keep your blood going to the right places at the right times, keeps you breathing, your heart at the right rate, your temperature regulated, and controls digestion (all the automatic stuff of the body that needs regulating but that you're generally unaware is happening). Dysautonomia means that these systems aren't working as they should.

Understanding how this dysfunctional system leads to symptoms can help make sense of both how you feel and why treatments work. When your autonomic nervous system isn't regulating blood flow properly, problems arise in two ways. First, there are direct effects from parts of your body not getting enough blood when and where they need it — for instance, your brain struggles to work properly when it isn't getting enough blood flow, and muscles tire

---

[1] Because we can never say things plainly and all love using Greek and Latin phrases. It does help a lot though having a common body of terms when working and communicating internationally.

quickly when they can't get enough oxygen[2]. Second, there are effects from your body trying to fix these blood flow problems — the brain not getting enough blood triggers emergency systems to try and get what it needs, resulting in complex effects including your heart racing to try to pump more blood and stress hormones rising to try to squeeze blood vessels and push blood where it's needed. You're running on emergency not because you're being chased by a tiger, but because you're trying to sit up. The body isn't meant to run on emergency all the time— it's exhausting. Treatments are generally aimed at improving this by first improving blood flow to places when it's needed as well as settling these emergency systems. This also helps explain why different people may need different approaches to treatment — some need help primarily with blood flow, others with moderating their body's response, and many need help with both.

Dysautonomia is the umbrella term covering all the different ways the autonomic nervous system (ANS) can go awry, much as if there was a term for "any kind of lung disease". Just as Heart failure is a term meaning "heart not working well enough to do what is required of it", but which doesn't tell you which of the many various ways the heart can be struggling is at work in a specific case.

The poster child of the Dysautonomias is Postural Orthostatic Tachycardia Syndrome[3] (POTS[4]). Classically, POTS presents in a tall, thin, young, hyper-flexible woman after an Epstein-Barr virus infection (aka glandular fever or infectious mononucleosis) with rapid heartbeat upon standing, dizziness, fatigue and potentially myriad other symptoms. However, the understanding has evolved, and we now recognise POTS across the lifespan — particularly in the COVID era. The COVID-19 pandemic has brought increased

---

[2] This is why many people with Dysautonomia feel short of breath despite having normal lung function — their brain and muscles aren't getting enough oxygen when they need it, which creates the same sensation as being out of breath from exercise.

[3] POTS is called a syndrome because it involves a collection of symptoms that commonly occur together, even though the underlying causes can vary between individuals.

[4] Distinct from Pott's disease which is tuberculosis of the spine, an important distinction if doing your own reading.

attention to Dysautonomia, as it appears to be a significant component of Long Covid syndrome for almost all sufferers.

POTS can affect anyone, regardless of age or gender. I've seen it develop after various infections including influenza, appendicitis, and cholecystitis. Sometimes, there's no apparent trigger at all — it "just happened". In older adults, POTS and other Dysautonomia symptoms are often mistaken for normal aging or other age-related conditions.

While the initial trigger may vary, practically, it doesn't really matter what caused it as we can't change the past.

The Dysautonomia's are mostly syndromes, rather than distinct diseases. A syndrome in medical terms is a grouping of symptoms that often go together. Often there can be a variety of causes or mechanisms, meaning that effective management (whether that be treating symptoms or the cause) can vary widely from person to person even though each individual presents with very similar issues.

This particular syndrome complex is often not considered by doctors. Despite having a long history with a variety of names[5], there is no blood test or imaging abnormality to prompt your doctors to think of it. If they don't think of it (having possibly never read that page in the textbook, or like me having been taught that it was very rare), then they are unlikely to specifically enquire about the symptoms and then arrange the appropriate testing, so it's very easy to miss. This leads to a lot of people being misdiagnosed, usually with conditions such as anxiety (as their

---

[5] Irritable heart syndrome: Described by physician Jacob Mendes Da Costa in 1871, resembling the modern concept of POTS.
Soldier's heart: Term coined by cardiologist Dr Thomas Lewis after WWI, as the condition was often found among military personnel.
Da Costa's syndrome: The condition came to be known by this name, now recognised as encompassing several distinct disorders including POTS.
Postural tachycardia syndrome: Coined in 1982 to describe a patient with postural tachycardia but not orthostatic hypotension.
Also, at varying times: neurocirculatory asthenia, mitral valve prolapse syndrome, hyperdynamic beta adrenergic state.
The term "Postural Orthostatic Tachycardia Syndrome", or POTS, was first used in 1993 by Dr's Ronald Schondorf and Phillip A. Low of the Mayo Clinic.

pulse is racing), depression (as they're tired and nothing else seems to be wrong), or an eating disorder (as it hurts or gives nausea when they eat so they don't want to). That doesn't mean that someone can't have more than one issue occurring at a time though. If there's any doubt, it's important to get an assessment from an appropriately trained professional to ensure that every part of your situation is managed effectively — your regular local doctor is best placed to help with this.

Worse yet, Dysautonomias often strike during crucial formative years when young people are building the foundations of their adult lives. Derailing education, delaying career development, and disrupting the normal social experiences and relationships that shape early adulthood. Every month spent waiting to find effective treatment represents missed opportunities and setbacks in this vital time of life. This is why I advocate for a more proactive approach to treatment, with careful but steady medication trials and dose adjustments, rather than the traditional "try this and come back in three months and we'll adjust things then" method. While safety remains paramount, there's no benefit in losing half a year or more just to work through a few medication trials that could be thoughtfully completed in a fraction of that time. The sooner we can help you feel better, the sooner you can get back to living your life.

Understanding vs. Managing Dysautonomia

While it's natural to want to understand exactly what's causing your symptoms, focusing too much on the underlying mechanisms can sometimes be counterproductive. Medical research frequently identifies differences between Dysautonomia patients and other people — unusual antibodies, altered blood flow patterns, or variations in nerve function. However, finding these differences in a particular individual rarely leads directly to new treatments. Even when we know what's different, often we can't safely target these changes with current technology, and there's no guarantee that addressing that one thing will fix the whole interlocking cascade of dysfunction (I wish biology was that simple).

What's most important is focusing on what we *can* change — the practical steps that help people feel and function better. The treatments in this guide have been proven to help, even though we don't always understand exactly why. Working with your healthcare team to systematically try established treatments is usually more productive than searching for a perfect explanation or pursuing elegant but theoretical solutions.

Remember: Healthcare providers aren't ignoring new research. They're focusing on providing approaches known to help while carefully evaluating new developments for practical benefit. The goal after all isn't to understand the myriad aspects of Dysautonomia — it's to help you feel better and get back to living your life.

Bridging the Gap: From Research to Treatment

This focus on practical management becomes even more important when we consider one of the most significant challenges in modern medicine — the lengthy delay between identifying potential treatments and implementing them effectively into routine clinical practice. This gap, often referred to as the "knowledge-to-practice gap" or "implementation gap", can span years or even decades, leaving many patients without access to potentially beneficial therapies.

Reasons for the Implementation Gap

- **Information Overload**: The sheer volume of medical research published annually makes it challenging for practitioners to stay current with all developments in their field.
- **Resistance to Change**: Established practices and treatment protocols can be difficult to modify, even in the face of new evidence.
- **Limited Resources**: Implementing new treatments often requires additional training, equipment, or staff, which may not be readily available in all healthcare settings.
- **Lack of Awareness**: Specialised knowledge often remains within niche communities of researchers and specialists, and takes time to reach general practitioners who see a wide variety of conditions.

- **Regulatory Hurdles**: The process of updating clinical guidelines and obtaining regulatory approvals can be lengthy and complex.
- **Economic Factors**: New treatments may be costly, and healthcare systems might be slow to adopt them due to budget constraints.

How This Guide Aims to Help

This guide on Dysautonomia management seeks to address this implementation gap in several ways:

- **Synthesising Current Knowledge**: By compiling the latest research and clinical experiences into a single, accessible resource, the aim is to make it easier for both patients and healthcare providers to access up-to-date information.
- **Practical Approach**: Rather than focusing on theory, this guide provides concrete, actionable steps for implementing effective treatments.
- **Bridging Specialties**: Dysautonomia often falls between multiple medical specialties. This guide brings together insights from various fields, helping to create a more comprehensive approach to care.
- **Patient Empowerment**: Providing patients with in-depth knowledge about their condition and treatment options hopefully enables them to have more informed and useful discussions with their healthcare providers.
- **Flexibility in Treatment**: The guide offers a range of treatment options and strategies, allowing for personalised care based on each patient's values and preferences, individual treatment responses, the resources available.
- **Ongoing Updates**: The current intention is to periodically update this guide to incorporate significant new research as the field evolves, helping to keep the information relevant.

By addressing these aspects, my hope is to play a small but significant role in bridging the gap between treatment development and implementation, ultimately improving care for individuals with Dysautonomia.

Why should you listen to me? (about the author)

I graduated from medical school in 1998 and am a proud Fellow of the Royal Australasian College of Physicians (FRACP), equivalent to specialist board certification in the United States. I am a General Internal Medicine Physician — a specialist non-specialist, having training in almost all the various sub-specialties of internal medicine, but not knowing any of them in the detail that a sub-specialist would. A specialist jack-of-all-trades but with an interest in bariatric medicine (the branch of medicine that deals with the study, prevention, and treatment of obesity and associated conditions). Most Dysautonomias are usually regarded as something best managed by a neurologist, with the specific condition of POTS frequently diagnosed and managed by a cardiologist. So why am I the one writing this?

I returned from Singapore to Australia in 2012, and at that time the local public health system wasn't hiring, so I established my own private practice. It had never occurred to me that a general physician in private medicine would get as many referrals for the assessment and management of fatigue as I was to receive[6].

General physicians often serve as "medical detectives", frequently receiving referrals for complex, undifferentiated conditions. Our broad training exposes us to a wide variety of medical issues and emphasises how multiple conditions can interact, hopefully equipping us to unravel these medical mysteries. This means we can often pinpoint the problem and save patients from a lengthy journey through multiple subspecialist appointments.

---

[6] Throughout this guide I share experiences from my clinical practice. Details have been carefully modified or combined from multiple cases, or presented as composite examples, to protect privacy while preserving educational value. Any resemblance to specific individuals is coincidental.

The first couple of "fatigued – please fix" referrals were an exercise in trying to come up on the spot with every possible thing that could make someone tired — which turns out to be a very long list. I soon realised that this was possibly going to be a significant part of my practice, so I sat down to list of all the things that could make someone tired. POTS and similar disorders were not on that list.

A few months later, a young woman was referred to me. She was otherwise well, but had severe fatigue and troublesome significant palpitations (in medical parlance meaning being aware of your heart beating), along with several other features. I admitted her to Coronary Care for close monitoring (suspecting an intermittent cardiac arrhythmia) and came around one morning to note that her pulse was in the high 80s beats per minute (bpm) while she was just lying calmly in the bed. This is a bit fast for an otherwise healthy young person at rest. Working through things I asked her a question and she jumped up out of the bed (unusual in coronary care) to look at her phone to get the answer and her pulse jumped to over 130 bpm on the monitor. This is not normal. "Wait, wait, wait. Forget what I asked you, lie back down again." The pulse went back to the high 80s bpm. I requested she stand up again and it went back above 130 bpm. It was all in a normal rhythm, just fast and excessively variable, and she actually did not feel too unwell at the time despite the very large rise.

I went to the computer, loaded an online textbook, thought "So this would be a....postural... tachycardia" and did a search. And up came Postural Orthostatic Tachycardia Syndrome. My next thought was, "What's that?", and the more I read about it, the more it seemed to fit her presentation.

I added Dysautonomia to the bottom of my causes of fatigue list and didn't expect to see it again soon, if ever.

Thinking back, I received probably 5 minutes, if that, on this topic in medical school back in the 1990s, which is not entirely surprising given the term was only first coined in 1993. Whilst it had been mentioned once or twice in my advanced training I had only seen 2 diagnosed cases in the years when I thought I wanted to be a cardiologist. With hindsight, particularly in Singapore, I think I missed several cases and I deeply regret that I likely told many young (mostly) women that they were just tired and need to sleep more as I could not find anything else going on.

As I consulted with people and worked through the list, I kept finding Dysautonomias. Day after day, week after week, to the point where I was diagnosing four or five new cases a week. Concerned I was over-diagnosing it, I sent patients for second opinions to respected senior cardiologists and neurologists around town. I half expected to be told I was wrong — instead, they agreed with my diagnoses and promptly sent the patients back to me for ongoing management, despite my expectation that they may take over their care.

Over the next few years, by word of mouth I ended up with a reputation for being the person to see if you thought you had one of these conditions and so I saw more and the cycle continued.

And then came COVID.... Dysautonomia is a big part of Long COVID (and Post-COVID-19 vaccination syndrome (PCVS) aka "Long Vax") and so far, the most treatable part of the syndrome, but instead of being limited largely to people under 25 years old at time of onset it's been right across the lifespan.

This guide is intended to share the lessons, tips and tricks I have learnt in the last 12 years. They don't always agree with the conventional approach, but it's what I've found to be the most effective way to help people one-on-one. The hope is that this will help sufferers, their families, friends and medical team to find a way to feel better sooner.

The plan is to update this document fairly frequently as new developments come along.

Who Should Use This Guide?

This guide is primarily intended for:

- **Patients with suspected or diagnosed Dysautonomia** who have been waiting for specialist care or have had limited treatment trials. Many individuals suffer for years without access to comprehensive care or having tried only a single first-line treatment. This guide aims to expedite diagnosis and initiate standard first-line therapies, potentially improving quality of life sooner.

- **Healthcare providers** who may be unfamiliar with Dysautonomia management but are caring for patients with these symptoms. This guide can serve as a resource to initiate appropriate diagnostic workups and treatment trials under medical supervision.

- **Family members and caregivers** of individuals with Dysautonomia, to better understand the condition and its management.

Who Should **Not** Rely Solely on This Guide?

- **Children under 14 years old**: As an adult medicine physician, my expertise and this guide's recommendations are tailored for individuals aged 14 and older. Paediatric Dysautonomia may require different approaches and should be managed by specialists in paediatric autonomic disorders.

- **Individuals over 55 years old with new-onset symptoms**: While Dysautonomia can occur at any age, new-onset symptoms in older adults warrant careful evaluation for other underlying conditions. These individuals should seek comprehensive medical assessment before applying the advice in this guide.

- **People with complex or atypical presentations**: Particularly those with features of Parkinsonism or symptoms beyond those described in this guide. These cases may indicate a distinct or coexisting condition that requires specialised evaluation and management.

- **Individuals with severe or life-threatening symptoms**: This guide is not a substitute for emergency medical care. Those experiencing severe symptoms should seek immediate medical attention.

- **Individuals with Parkinson's Disease**: While orthostatic hypotension is a common dysautonomia in Parkinson's Disease, sufferers should work with their neurologist for management, as they require different therapeutic approaches than described here.

Important Considerations Before Starting

- Dysautonomia can coexist with other medical conditions. While the treatments outlined here may often overlap with management strategies for related disorders, this is not always the case.

- This guide is intended to complement, not replace, professional medical care. Always consult with a healthcare provider before initiating or changing any treatment regimen.

- If symptoms persist or worsen despite following the recommendations in this guide, further medical evaluation is necessary to rule out other conditions or complications.

How to Use This Guide

This guide is designed to be both comprehensive and accessible. You don't need to read it cover-to-cover — feel free to focus on the sections most relevant to you right now and come back to others as needed.

To help you understand the medical terminology used throughout:

- A comprehensive glossary is provided at the back of the book where you can look up any unfamiliar terms,
- Complex medical concepts are explained in plain language where possible, and
- Examples and analogies are used to help explain difficult concepts.

The guide includes several practical resources after the main section:

- Lists of useful organisations and websites,
- Treatment summaries and protocols, and
- Letter templates for various situations.

These resources are also available online at http://aionhealth.com.au/dysautonomia-resources in printable format for easy use.

Remember — while there are many shared features, everyone's experience with Dysautonomia is different. Use this guide as a resource to help inform discussions with your healthcare team rather than as a replacement for personalised medical advice.

Diagnosis

Key Points

- Dysautonomia affects the body's automatic control systems (heart rate, blood pressure, temperature).
- Diagnosis based on:
  - Pattern of typical symptoms,
  - Changes in heart rate/blood pressure on standing,
  - Home measurements over a week,
  - Excluding other medical causes.
- Treatment may help even if not meeting the strict criteria.

So, how does one diagnose Dysautonomia? There are many, many ways a complicated structure such as the autonomic nervous system can malfunction, including:

- Neurogenic orthostatic hypotension (nOH) where there is a large drop in blood pressure without a pulse rate change (which can exist by itself or be associated with another condition such as Parkinson's disease),
- Vasovagal syncope (also known as neurally mediated syncope or sometimes called neurocardiogenic syncope),
- Chronic isolated orthostatic intolerance, and
- Postural Orthostatic Tachycardia Syndrome, or POTS (of which there are subtypes).

I have moved away from the conventional tilt table test as the diagnostic test of choice, as it can be hard to access and is relatively costly, has a frustratingly high false negative rate (appears to miss it), and also the potential to overcall things. Instead, I request lying blood pressure and pulse rate followed by a standing blood pressure and pulse rate twice a day, morning and night, for a week in the home environment. This is distinct from the vast majority of recommendations, which recommend either a Tilt Table Test, the more complicated Active Standing Test, or the NASA Lean Test, in that it does not have specified times to do the standing blood pressure and pulse. As long as the test works, I prefer to keep it simple and some people with a severe case can't stand long enough to do some varieties of these tests.

I have found this to be a very useful way to help make the diagnosis. By taking a number of readings over time, we reduce the effect of random variability from day to day in a condition that can vary significantly. The finding of an abnormal Blood Pressure (BP) response to standing, or more often an abnormal Pulse Rate (PR) response to standing, in conjunction with a suggestive history and having excluded all other causes, has been a very useful approach.

When you stand up, normally the large blood vessels in your body rapidly constrict, maintaining blood flow to the head. This typically results in a small rise in blood pressure, while the pulse rate either stays the same or also increases slightly (by definition, normally less than 20 bpm). However, after performing this test on many (many) people in various settings over the last decade, I've found that in healthy young people, the pulse rate typically only increases by 0-10 bpm — unless there is something significant going on, like severe dehydration or sepsis.

This is relevant because the current diagnostic criteria for POTS in someone under the age of 20 years old is a postural tachycardia (how much the pulse rate increases on standing up) of greater than 40 bpm, and in someone 20 years old or older by a rise of greater than 30 bpm. They don't have to meet it every time, but an abnormal pattern does suggest something is going on. This leaves us with a problem. If someone does not meet this cut off, then do you not treat them? What if someone has a very suggestive story that only goes up 28 or 29 beats per minute? Do you tell them to go away and come back when it's 30 bpm or over? I suggest that it is still worth a treatment trial, even if it is instead labelled "Dysautonomia not meeting POTS criteria" or "Orthostatic intolerance".

What matters in a day-to-day clinical setting is less "What exactly should we call it?" and more "How can we help?" (unless dealing with insurance companies or governmental bodies — they love labels). That then raises the question, what about a rise of 29 bpm? What about 28? 27? 25?

I have on occasion, and with a great deal of clarification that I am not certain that this will help, tried treating people with a good story, no other apparent cause, and a postural tachycardia of as low as 17 bpm. Most of these cases improved significantly. The definition with hard cut-offs was derived for the purposes of research studies where you do have to draw a line somewhere on who definitely has the condition versus who definitely does not. The clinical practice of medicine though is about trying to help, even when something isn't as clear cut as we may wish. Sometimes the only way to do that is to at least see if something (safe and cheap) works rather than not even trying at all.

It is also probably wise to get a 24-hour Holter monitor and strongly consider a transthoracic echocardiogram to exclude possibly serious heart conditions such as supraventricular tachycardia or a structural cardiac abnormality.

Similarly, it is important to exclude other treatable conditions presenting with fatigue, which is why I keep Dysautonomia at the end of my fatigue screen, and often people do have more than one thing going on.

One condition that is easily confused with a Dysautonomia is Myalgic Encephalomyelitis/Chronic Fatigue Syndrome (ME/CFS)[7]. The ME/CFS diagnostic criteria[8] actually include "Orthostatic intolerance — Worsening of symptoms upon assuming and maintaining upright posture. Symptoms are improved, although not necessarily abolished, by lying back down or elevating the feet."

---

[7] ME and CFS are two names for the same condition, now commonly referred to as ME/CFS in medical literature and by health organisations
[8] 2015 Institute of Medicine diagnostic criteria for ME/CFS

This leads to a decision — do you treat it as ME/CFS or as a Dysautonomia? We have a lot more treatment options for Dysautonomias than we do for ME/CFS. So, in my experience, it's better to try treating as Dysautonomia first and seeing if it helps, instead of jumping straight to a ME/CFS diagnosis and potentially missing out on effective treatments.

It's interesting — when I watched old footage of ME/CFS support groups, I spotted many folks with signs of what we now recognise as POTS or similar conditions. It really makes you wonder how many people might have been misdiagnosed or missed out on potential treatments in the past.

So, my approach is this: Let's explore the Dysautonomia angle first. If it turns out that's not the whole picture, we can always circle back to managing it as ME/CFS. But at least we've given ourselves the best shot at finding effective treatments.

Red Flags: When to Consider Alternative Diagnoses and Specialist Referral

While Dysautonomia is often a benign condition in that it doesn't kill but rather just makes you miserable, certain symptoms or findings should prompt further investigation and specialist referral.

Seek Emergency Care if experiencing:

- **True Syncope on Exertion**: Fainting or feeling like you are going to faint during physical activity (not just upon standing) may indicate a serious cardiac condition, or
- Chest pain accompanied by shortness of breath, particularly with exertion, or
- Severe, sudden-onset neurological symptoms like confusion, difficulty speaking, or weakness on one side.

Specialist Medical Review Needed If:

- **Family History of Cardiomyopathy or Sudden Death especially under 40 years old**: This could suggest an inherited heart condition.
- **Abnormal ECG findings, including**:
  - Significant arrhythmias,
  - Prolonged QT interval,
  - Brugada pattern, or
  - Other concerning conduction abnormalities.
- **Abnormal echocardiogram**: Any structural heart abnormalities warrant further cardiac evaluation.
- **Signs of more generalised autonomic failure**, such as:
  - New bladder or bowel dysfunction,
  - Complete inability to sweat, or
  - Severe blood pressure fluctuations.

If any of these red flags are present, prompt referral to a cardiologist or neurologist is recommended for comprehensive evaluation. The presence of red flags doesn't rule out Dysautonomia, but it may indicate the need to investigate other conditions or complications.

Treatments

Key Points

Treatment aims:

- Exercise is currently the only proven way to speed recovery.
- Other treatments help manage symptoms.
- Most people need multiple approaches.

Core management includes:

- Structured exercise program,
- Careful fluid intake,
- Salt supplementation,
- Compression garments, and
- Mental health support.

Treatment plans:

- Individually tailored,
- Regularly reviewed, and
- Adjusted as needed.

So, having excluded other causes, and thinking it's worth a treatment trial to see if someone feels better, what do you do?

One thing I've found in the last decade is that — no matter what the books say — everyone is different and sometimes the only way to see if something will help someone is to try it and see.

People with Dysautonomia also seem to be prone to having unusual side effects, so it's best to <u>start low and go slow</u>, but importantly to <u>actually try</u> — because if you don't try, you're never sure if it could have helped.

It's important to explicitly recognise that these symptoms are very real, even when blood tests and x-rays come back normal. Having normal test results doesn't mean your symptoms are "just psychological" (more on that later).

I also provide references to various useful online resources to see if the and information and stories there resonate with their experience (listed at the end of this guide).

Next, I emphasise that this is a condition that generally does get better as we almost never[9] see it in people 40 to 50+ years old. Unfortunately, it can take years to improve spontaneously. Treatment is aimed at shortening that recovery time and helping the person to feel better and more functional in the meantime.

Exercise

To that end, the **only thing that has been demonstrated to improve recovery time** is a certain type of exercise program[10]. I know — if you're struggling to even stand up or do basic daily tasks, the word "exercise" probably makes you want to stop reading right now. But stick with me, because this isn't about going for a run or hitting the gym.

When we talk about exercise for Dysautonomia, we're starting exactly where you are — even if that's lying flat in bed. For some people, initial reconditioning might be just 15 seconds of moving your arms while lying down. That's okay. The key is finding your starting point and building up gradually from there.

For a while, I gave detailed exercise advice, but soon realised something important: it's really hard to teach individualised,

---

[9] Well, at least we didn't until Long Covid.
[10] Unfortunately, there are 2 situations that are exceptions to this. The hyperadrenergic variant of POTS doesn't appear to respond well to exercise, and people with severe hypermobility often need to dedicate their exercise time to minimising complications and injuries resulting from that as a priority. In neither case though will regular, tailored, appropriate exercise hurt though — it just may not help treat the Dysautonomia specifically as much as we would like.

complex exercise programs with multiple contingencies in a few minutes. This resulted in some pushing themselves too hard, while others would be too cautious. Neither approach was ideal. That's why I now strongly recommend working with an Accredited Exercise Physiologist (EP) who understands Dysautonomia[11]. They're trained to help you find the right balance — challenging your system enough to improve, but not so much that you crash. Working with an EP allows for careful monitoring and adjustment of your exercise program based on your individual response.

Think of it as retraining your autonomic nervous system. The exercise stresses your system just enough that it has to learn to do its job better, but not so much that it gets overwhelmed. It's a delicate balance, and that's why having professional guidance is so valuable.

If you can manage this without medications — great. But many people need medication to be able to exercise meaningfully without flaring their symptoms. If medications help you both feel better in general and also to engage more meaningfully with exercise, that's a win, because exercise is what's going to help you get better in the long run.

So, whilst exercising with a Dysautonomia can be challenging, it's an important part of managing the condition. Here are some key principles to keep in mind:

1. Start Slowly: Begin with low-intensity, horizontal exercises like swimming, or floor work, or using a reclined exercise bike. Gradually increase the duration and intensity over time.

2. Consistency: Aim for regular exercise, ideally 30 minutes of moderate activity on most days of the week — though almost no one can manage to start at this level. Consistency helps improve cardiovascular fitness and muscle strength.

3. Hydration: Stay well-hydrated (and well salt-loaded) before, during, and after exercise to help manage

---

[11] Many physiotherapists also now have similar training — "thanks" Covid.

symptoms. Hydration powders are recommended. Whichever one you like and tolerate (see treatment section on fluid and salt loading).

4. <u>Listen to Your Body</u>: Pay attention to how you feel and adjust your exercise routine accordingly. Avoid overexertion and take breaks as needed. It is normal to feel a bit fatigued after exercising, but if you crash for the next few days after a session, then you overdid it.

5. <u>Expect Variability</u>: How much you can manage will likely change from day to day and week to week (hopefully improving on average). Just because something was too much one session doesn't mean that will always be the case — just cut it back a bit the next time and reassess. Also, if you do happen to overdo it and crash, whilst not ideal, it won't hurt your progress in the long run.

6. <u>Timing</u>: Be flexible as you will likely find that you manage the exercise better and have better results by doing it at the time of day when you're feeling at your best (most energetic/least symptomatic), whether it's after fluid and salt loading and/or medications or just a good time for you.

7. <u>Strength Training</u>: You don't want Dysautonomia and to be deconditioned as well. Incorporate strength training, especially for the legs and core, to improve muscle pump function and overall stability.

8. <u>Gradual Progression</u>: Increase exercise duration and intensity **very** gradually to avoid triggering symptoms. Of course, the only way to progress is to try a bit more at times. Be guided by your EP.

9. <u>Body Position</u>: Start with exercises that keep you in a flat position, then progress to a recumbent, then eventually a seated position and slowly progress to more upright activities.

An exercise physiologist I work closely with currently recommends an approach promoted in a 2021 research paper[12] as a good place to start, which he then tailors to the individual.

It is designed to gradually improve symptoms and function over time. It's important to note that you may initially feel a bit worse for up to 6 weeks after starting this program. This is normal and usually improves with consistent effort.

However, listen to your body and stop if you experience severe discomfort or unusual symptoms. If you crash afterwards then the intensity in that session was probably too much and you'll need to back off a bit next time.

1. **Start with gentle conditioning exercises:**

- Week 1: Begin with 10 minutes of reclined exercises such as:
    - Recumbent cycling at a very light intensity,
    - Floor-based resistance exercises,
    - Gentle walking (if tolerated) with frequent rest breaks.
- Each subsequent week: Try to add 3–5 minutes to your total exercise time.
- Goal: Build up to 30–45 minutes of exercise that you can tolerate without crashing. This will likely take months to achieve.
- Progress from lying to reclined to upright positions as tolerated.
- Remember: What counts as "exercise" will vary greatly between individuals, especially at the start.

Note: The intensity will be determined individually based on what you can reasonably achieve. Don't push yourself too hard, especially at the beginning.

---

[12] Christopher H. Gibbons, Gustavo Silva, Roy Freeman. Cardiovascular exercise as a treatment of postural orthostatic tachycardia syndrome: A pragmatic treatment trial. Heart Rhythm, 2021;18(8): 1361-1368. doi: 10.1016/j.hrthm.2021.01.017

2. Resistance Training:

- Your exercise physiologist will help with maintaining correct form and preventing injury. This is particularly important for people with hypermobility.
- Starting recommendation:
  - 1–2 days per week, separated by at least one rest day,
  - 10–20 minutes per session.
- Long-term goal: Build towards 2 sessions per week of 30–45 minutes.
- Exercise routine:
  - Perform 2 sets of 10 repetitions of each exercise.
  - For the second set, do as many repetitions as you can manage comfortably.
  - Recommended exercises:
    - Seated leg press,
    - Leg curl,
    - Leg extension,
    - Calf raise,
    - Chest press,
    - Gentle abdominal exercises,
    - Side planks or Pilates-based floor exercises,
    - Seated row.

Note: Start with body weight or very light weights. Only increase weight when you can consistently perform more than 10 repetitions with good form and without post-exercise crashes.

3. Swimming: An Ideal Exercise for Dysautonomia

- An excellent form of exercise for Dysautonomia management, offering major benefits such as:
  - being able to be done whilst horizontal, with
  - the water squeezing on you, and
  - helping to regulate heat.

- Again, this is best guided by a professionally trained expert familiar with Dysautonomia management.
- Starting recommendation:
  - Begin with short sessions (5–10 minutes) a few times a week and gradually increase duration as tolerated.
  - Start with gentle exercises like water walking or floating before progressing to swimming strokes.
  - Use flotation devices if needed to feel more secure in the water.
  - Focus on relaxed breathing to help manage any anxiety associated with exercise.
- Swimming Techniques
  - Water Walking: Start in chest-deep water and walk forward, backward, and sideways. This is a great way to begin if full swimming is initially too challenging.
  - Floating and Treading Water: Practice floating on your back or treading water to improve comfort in the water and work on breath control.
  - Gentle Strokes: Begin with easy strokes like breaststroke or sidestroke, which keep your head above water and allow for easier breathing.
  - Interval Training: As you progress, try alternating between periods of gentle swimming and rest to gradually build endurance.
- Safety Considerations
  - Always swim with a buddy or in a supervised pool.
  - Stay hydrated and listen to your body — exit the pool if you feel dizzy or overly fatigued.
  - When exiting the pool, sit on the edge for 1–2 minutes before standing up to allow your body to adjust.

o   And again, **consult with your exercise physiologist** before starting a swimming program and as you improve.

Remember: Start slow and progress at your own pace. It's normal to have good days and bad days. Consistency is key, but always prioritise your safety and comfort.

All treatments other than exercise are aimed at feeling better and being more able to engage with life, but these will not fix the underlying problem.

There is no single magic formula, and it will take some trial and error. Don't give up due to one bad session.

With time the expectation is to feel better, which will hopefully enable better engagement with physical rehabilitation leading to more rapid improvement in mood and outlook as well as function.

Things that will potentially help you feel better (symptomatic therapies)

Fluid loading:

Most people have already worked this out. I call it "water bottle sign" — if someone walks in carrying a water bottle and has been referred for fatigue it's extremely likely they have a Dysautonomia.

The guidelines call for 3+ litres a day, the problem of course being that the kidneys down under the bottom ribs don't care what's going on up at the head and see all this extra fluid and promptly do what kidneys do with too much fluid. Which ends up with people going to the toilet all the time. More on this later.

Salt loading:

The guidelines call for 8g+ of salt a day from all sources. This is very unusual advice from a doctor (MORE salt?!), but for the short term and given most people with Dysautonomias have problematically low blood pressure (BP) it's not an issue. If you are one in the minority with high or borderline high BP, then skip this part.

Do NOT shake out 8g of salt into your hand from the salt shaker and swallow it — you'll just vomit.

Most practitioners recommend getting a lot of salt in the form of food. But there's a limit to how many anchovy, olive, cheese and ham sandwiches you can eat in day. Feel free to add salt to food (not chips — my bariatric physician side can't recommend that), and if that isn't enough, try supplements.

Interestingly a lot of people with Dysautonomia feel better after a few litres of intravenous (IV) saline. For reference a litre of normal saline contains 9g of salt. People in hospital wards on IV fluids would not uncommonly have 3 litres per day containing 27 grams of salt, straight into their veins, and it can be given a lot quicker. For people in this situation, it's "More salt, more often" — the trick is keeping it palatable and what the gut can handle.

In capsules for supplementation there are salt (NaCl) and sodium bicarbonate (NaHCO$_3$) available. Sodium bicarbonate (baking soda) is usually better tolerated by the stomach, but do NOT eat straight baking soda, and best not to have more than a few of these a day without consulting with a doctor. A wide variety of electrolyte replacement drinks and supplements are also available, such as those for marathons or triathlons. Feel free to use whichever one you like and which works for you, though best to avoid the ones high in sugar.

Intravenous saline is not recommended as a standard therapy and I only consider it when everything else has failed, particularly given the practical difficulties and risks in the non-hospital setting. That said, it can be an effective emergency rescue therapy for a bad flare, or if someone has to be at the top of their game for a special occasion e.g. an examination or wedding.

Compression:

I recommend the higher and tighter the better. Usually this means waist high stockings in the grade 2 (22–30mmHg) compression range. Less than that usually isn't as useful as you'd wish and tighter than that isn't bearable. The most important areas to compress are the thighs, buttocks and abdomen — up to the knees just isn't enough.

Unfortunately, the scientifically studied compression garments are quite thick and not terribly warm weather friendly (the time they are usually needed the most) nor very fashionable, but the spandex/elastane ones do seem to work, are much better tolerated and are a lot more fashion forward, with the downside being that they generally (not always) cost significantly more. If you find some inexpensive compression garments that meet the criteria above (waist-high, grade 2 compression), they're worth trying. While they may have issues with heat and might wear out quickly, using them can help determine if compression is beneficial for you before investing in more expensive pairs.

Some people find that abdominal compression alone can provide significant relief, especially when longer compression garments are too warm. When using an abdominal binder, it's important to ensure that it's snug but not so tight that it impairs breathing or causes discomfort.

How to use: they only work if you're wearing them. If you can only tolerate them for shorter periods to start with, do that and gradually increase as tolerated.

Tip: These are particularly useful if worn during a trip (flights or long car/train trips) and can prevent the flares that usually go along with these.

Psychology:

Being unwell is stressful personally and will place a strain on relationships. Having someone to talk to who isn't a friend or family can be very useful and I strongly recommend that, if possible, people meet regularly with a trained psychologist. Even if it's just to discuss how this isn't how you want life to be.

As previously mentioned, many young people (especially women) are commonly misdiagnosed with:

- anxiety ("You're a young healthy person with palpitations, you must be anxious"),

- depression ("You're tired all the time and your blood tests are normal. You must be depressed"), or

- an eating disorder ("You don't want to eat because it makes you feel worse. You must have an eating disorder"), or

- Functional Neurological Disorder (FND) ("Your symptoms don't fit a clear traditional neurological pattern, and your tests are normal, so it must be functional")[13].

That doesn't mean that you can't have more than one issue at the same time though. If there's any doubt, it's important to get an

---

[13] It can be hard for the brain to function normally when not getting enough blood. It's worth noting the FND diagnostic criteria and the POTS criteria are quite distinct and they have **not** been found to be commonly associated so far.

assessment from a trained professional to ensure that every part of your situation is managed effectively.

A relationship with a psychologist is a very personal thing and if you don't feel rapport with the person you're seeing that's fine and will be understood. That doesn't mean support isn't for you, it means that you haven't found the right fit yet. It's very common for people to see 3 to 5 psychologists before they find the right person for them. GPs, national organisations[14], and online searches are all good ways to find someone to try.

Co-existing conditions

People can have two (or more) problems at the same time, and so any conditions associated with fatigue should also be checked for and addressed if present. Two common ones are:

- Iron insufficiency, particularly if menstruation is occurring, or

- Low Vitamin C levels, due to gastrointestinal citrus intolerance.

There are also conditions that seem to be intrinsically linked to Dysautonomia through shared mechanisms or predispositions — such as hypermobility, MCAS, ADHD, autism spectrum disorder, migraines, and endometriosis. These will be discussed in detail in the Associated Conditions section later in this guide.

Both groups of conditions should be identified and appropriately managed alongside the Dysautonomia for best results.

---

[14] in Australia: http://psychology.org.au/find-a-psychologist

Supplements and dietary interventions

A (very) wide variety of supplements have been tried by various patients I've seen over the years, whether recommended by friends, family, the internet, or naturopaths. Unfortunately, none have been successful, at least not enough for anyone to stick with any of them long-term.

It would seem to go without saying, but when coming across things online (or anywhere) it's always worth considering whether the person promising something has a financial interest in making a sale. One strength of modern medicine (at least the Australian system) is that a physician has nothing to gain by prescribing one treatment over another. We get paid by the patient for providing expert advice — not because one treatment has a better financial margin over another. If it is effective and is safe, doctors will recommend it.

That said, if you do want to try something, just as with the medications after this, it's probably wise to start low and go slow. If it helps, has no or manageable side effects, and the cost is reasonable — great! If it doesn't work, then maybe don't buy another supply.

Important Note About Treatment Options

Looking at all these treatment options might feel overwhelming at first — that's completely normal. Remember that you don't need to tackle everything at once.

The goal is to work through options one step at a time, at your own pace, in partnership with your healthcare team. Starting with the basics (like staying well hydrated, trying compression garments and gradually building up exercise tolerance), gives you a foundation to build on.

From there, you and your doctor can thoughtfully explore which medications or other treatments might help you feel better. There's no race to try everything, and what works best for you may be different from what works for someone else.

Medications

Important: The information in this guide is for educational purposes only. Always consult with your healthcare provider before starting, stopping, or changing any medication regimen.

Regulatory Notice: Many medications[15] discussed in this guide are prescribed "off-label" for Dysautonomia in Australia, meaning they are being used in ways not officially approved by the Therapeutic Goods Administration (TGA)[16]. This is common practice for rare or emerging conditions, but requires careful consideration by prescribing physicians. International readers should note that:

- Medication availability varies by country,
- Regulatory approvals differ between jurisdictions,
- Local prescribing guidelines may vary,
- Insurance coverage for off-label use varies significantly, and
- Always consult local healthcare providers about medication availability and approval status in your jurisdiction.

Summaries about each of the medications and their use is also available in streamlined handout form at the end of this guide. This information is for both your usage and for sharing with your regular medical practitioner, who may not be as familiar with these agents in managing Dysautonomia.

---

[15] All product names, trademarks, and registered trademarks mentioned in this guide are the property of their respective owners. The use of these names and trademarks is for identification purposes only and does not imply endorsement of any specific brand, product, or company over others.
[16] The Australian equivalent of the US Food and Drug Administration (FDA), or the European Medicines Agency (EMA).

Key Points

Medication approach:

- Start low and increase slowly,
- Focus on symptom improvement,
- Monitor for side effects, and
- Adjust based on response.

Treatment strategy:

- Try one medication at a time, and
- Find the lowest effective dose, and
- Add others if needed, and
- Regular review.

Success measured by:

- Feeling better,
- Improved function, and
- Manageable side effects.

In the interest of timely and efficient therapy, I've found it more effective to provide protocols on how to gradually increase the dosages to find the optimal level for each individual, rather than simply saying, "Try half a tablet of this twice a day, and I'll see you in three months", as neither the patient nor I have time to waste in finding an effective treatment. This approach has proven to be both safe and effective for over a decade.

Unfortunately, whilst we'd like to be able to say "you have this variant of this condition, so this is the treatment and it'll work", which is often the case and is great in many fields of medicine, Dysautonomia doesn't seem to work that way.

Even the seemingly clearest cases of one subtype (e.g. hypovolaemic or hyperadrenergic POTS) don't always respond to the treatment that they're "supposed to". I wish biology was that easy.

For instance, I saw two sisters, both with hypermobility (loose- or double-jointed), both severely affected by their symptoms (each initially requiring a wheelchair). One responded well to pyridostigmine (an agent that increases synaptic acetylcholine levels) at high dose. Given their close relationship, when I saw her sister soon after, I thought "Great, I know what to do here", but pyridostigmine did very little. After further trials she most benefited from a large dose of fludrocortisone (a synthetic mineralocorticoid). Despite having the same symptoms, the same pattern of postural tachycardia and BP drop, and being so closely related, their treatments were very different. Patients don't always read the textbook and behave as it says.

Also, dosing can be completely different. I've had people make huge steps forward with as little as 25 micrograms (mcg) fludrocortisone a day, whilst I've read about people taking as much as 40 times (=1000mcg) that.

So, the principle is — start low, go slow and see if it helps and is tolerated. If you get benefit before side effects — great! If the side effects kick in first — stop it and try something else. It's just not the therapy for you.

It's not about treating numbers on a page (e.g. the amount of postural tachycardia day by day) either — it's about feeling better. They're also conditions that vary, with "better" and "worse" days. The goal is feeling better on a good day and having more good days, with fewer bad days and which are not as debilitating (hopefully so you can get into the exercise more to progressively improve baseline unmedicated function). The key is to pause every few weeks to thoughtfully reflect on these trends — what's improved, what hasn't, and how your overall function has changed[17].

---

[17] While detailed symptom diaries may seem helpful, they often lead to excessive focus on daily fluctuations. Taking time every few weeks to reflect on overall trends typically provides more meaningful insight into progress.

Currently there are no Australian Therapeutic Goods Administration (TGA), or Pharmaceutical Benefits Scheme (PBS) listed medications for any form of Dysautonomia. As such all medications are prescribed "off-label" (using a medication in a way that hasn't been officially approved by the government agency responsible for regulating drugs and medical products) as is common for what are considered unusual conditions. I can't speak to the regulatory framework in any other country, so this will need to be discussed with the local prescribing doctor. They are all prescription only medications here.

General Medication Management Principles

Key Principles:

1. **Start Low, Go Slow**: Begin with a low dose and gradually increase until you find the minimum effective dose (as per the described protocols).
2. **Aim for Improvement**: The goal is to feel better, not worse. If a medication consistently makes you feel worse, it may not be the right fit — stop it.
3. **Be Patient**: Give each medication a fair chance to work. It may take time to see the full effects.
4. **Monitor Your Progress**: Keep track of your symptoms and how they change with medication.
5. **Communicate with Your Doctor**: Regularly update your healthcare provider about your experiences.

Understanding "Better" vs "Worse"

- **Better Days**: More energy, fewer symptoms, improved quality of life.
- **Worse Days**: Increased fatigue, more severe symptoms, difficulty with daily activities.

Remember: Dysautonomia's are conditions of ups and downs. A "bad day" shortly after starting a new medication doesn't necessarily mean the medication is what is causing problems. Look for overall trends in your symptoms over time.

When to cease a medication trial and inform your doctor:

- If you consistently feel worse after starting a medication, or
- If you experience new or unexpected symptoms.

When to consider pausing a medication trial:

- If other factors are complicating the picture (like an acute infection, hormonal changes, weather changes, travel, lack of sleep, stress, or changes to your routine/activity level) — it's okay to pause and try again when things are more stable.
- If you're unsure about changes in your condition — you can always stop or pause things, discuss the situation with your doctor, and potentially retry the medication later.

Remember: The goal is to feel better — if you don't then stop the medication and discuss other options with your prescribing doctor.

Medication Selection Based on Likely Subvariant:

The individual order of trialling these is best discussed based on your exact circumstances with your prescribing doctor.

Most people will need a combination of agents, finding that two agents at a lower dose are more effective or are better tolerated than just one at a high dose. Finding the right combination is just a matter of working things through and finding what works for any individual case.

When initiating treatment for Dysautonomia, the choice of medication often depends on the predominant symptoms and likely subvariant. Here's a general guide:

- **Significant Pre-syncope/Syncope, postural drop in BP, or elevated serum albumin:**
  1. Start with: Fludrocortisone.
  2. Rationale: Helps increase blood volume and improve orthostatic tolerance.

- **Resting tachycardia (75+ bpm) or rapid rise with minimal exertion:**
    1. Start with: Beta-blockers (e.g. propranolol, bisoprolol, nebivolol) or Ivabradine.
    2. Rationale: Helps control heart rate and reduce palpitations.
- **Significant Fatigue with Normal/Low Heart Rate, or prominent constipation:**
    1. Start with: Pyridostigmine.
    2. Rationale: May improve energy levels without excessively raising heart rate.
- **Prominent Vasodilation or Blood Pooling:**
    1. Start with: Midodrine.
    2. Rationale: Helps constrict blood vessels and improve blood return to the heart.

Remember, these are general guidelines. Individual responses frequently vary, and a combination of medications is often necessary for optimal symptom control.

Agents taken regularly (to make the average quality of life better):

Fludrocortisone (Florinef): keep refrigerated but not frozen.

How it works: A synthetic mineralocorticoid. Tells the kidneys to hold onto sodium (salt), which then holds onto water. To hold onto sodium, they must discard something else — potassium.

> **Note:** Potassium loss is very rarely an issue with doses up to about 300mcg (3 tablets) a day unless on a very unusual diet.

Dosage forms: There is only one formulation: 100mcg (0.1mg) tablets, which are scored down the middle, to ease their being divided in half. Keep refrigerated.

Usual side effects: Uncomfortable fluid retention, bloating, headache, stomach ache.

How to take: Increase every 5–7 days until "better" or side effects. If any of these side effects (or anything else that seems bad) develop → stop. Once better go back onto whatever was the last "best dose" (whatever gave most improvement without side effects).

If your best dose was none, then this isn't the one for you and it's time to try something else on the list.

Standard protocol:

- ½ tablet (50mcg) per day for a week and assess — if feeling great stop at this level, if no difference or a bit better but you'd like to see if a higher dose helps more, then increase to:

- 1 tablet (100mcg) per day for a week and reassess — if feeling great stop at this level, if no difference or a bit better but you'd like to see if a higher dose helps more, then increase to:

- 1 ½ tablets (150mcg) per day for a week and reassess — if feeling great stop at this level, if no difference or a bit better but you'd like to see if a higher dose helps more, then increase to:

- 2 tablets (200mcg) per day for a week and reassess — if feeling great stop at this level, if no difference or a bit better but you'd like to see if a higher dose helps more, then increase to:

- 2 ½ tablets (250mcg) per day for a week and reassess — if feeling great stop at this level, if no difference or a bit better but you'd like to see if a higher dose helps more, then increase to:

- 3 tablets (300mcg) per day for a week and reassess — if feeling great stop at this level, if no difference since starting — give up.

- Discuss with a doctor (who will probably check your blood potassium level) before going past this dose.

- I **strongly recommend** careful monitoring of serum potassium (a blood test) levels if you go past this as many people will need specific potassium supplementation to avoid the potential complications of low potassium. It is not uncommon that people do feel better on even higher doses — but it does need more careful monitoring.

Again, if you get side effects, then skip a dose or 2 until recovered then go back to whatever dose worked best for you.

Beta-blockers:

- **Propranolol (Inderal or Deralin)** 10mg tablets **or**

- **Bisoprolol (Bicor)** 5mg tablets **or**

- **Atenolol (Noten)** 50mg tablets **or**

- **another** (there are quite a few different agents in this class)[18].

Beta-blockers (β-blockers) are a very cheap and well-known class of medications every doctor will be familiar with as they are commonly used to treat various heart conditions, high blood pressure, and anxiety. In Dysautonomia, they can help manage symptoms by slowing the heart rate and potentially improving blood pressure regulation. The usual side effect is to drop the blood pressure which sounds like a bad idea, but in POTS there is often an opposite effect.

If at any stage you feel notably worse in any way, stop taking it, and discuss with your treating practitioner. The idea is to feel better not worse after all.

Once settled, consider going back to whatever dose you felt best at. If the best dose was none, then this treatment isn't the one for you and it's time to try something else on the list.

---

[18] A note on beta-blocker selection: While there are numerous beta-blockers available, and some research suggests certain ones may work better for specific POTS subtypes, choosing between them is a complex clinical decision requiring careful consideration of many factors. Rather than attempting to detail all these various factors in this introductory guide, I've focused on the most commonly used options. The key is finding what works for you through careful trials, rather than getting too focused on theoretical matches between subtypes and specific medications. Your doctor is best placed to help determine which beta-blocker might be most appropriate to try first based on your specific situation.

Usual side effects: Include apathy, nightmares, erectile dysfunction and excessive slowing of the heart. Dizziness on standing is a common effect for these agents normally, but in Dysautonomia there is often a paradoxical improvement in these symptoms. Despite the benefits beta-blockers can reduce blood volume further which can be a concern in hypovolemic patients (people where the condition is running their body dry compared to where it should be).

Standard Protocols:

Propranolol

Advantages: Well studied in POTS, cheap, often reduces the frequency of migraines.

Disadvantages: Can interact with some ADHD medications, potentially making them less effective.

Dosage forms: 10mg tablets, or 40mg tablets if a higher dose is needed.

How to take: Start with one 10mg tablet in the morning and one at night. Increase every 3–5 days as follows until finding the right dose for you:

Morning	Night	
1	1	for 3 or more days, then
2	2	for 3 or more days, then
3	3	for 3 or more days, then
4	4	for 3 or more days.

If not helping by here → stop taking.

Discuss with a doctor before going past this dose, but I have had rare patients go (much) higher than this to properly get things under control.

Bisoprolol

Advantages: Cheap, doesn't get into the brain well so doesn't negatively interact with ADHD medications and less apathy and nightmares, only once a day for most people.

Disadvantages: Not as well studied in POTS. Won't help migraine.

Dosage forms: 2.5mg, 5mg and 10mg tablets

How to take: Start with ½ a 5mg tablet (=2.5mg) twice a day. Increase every 3 to 5 days until finding the right dose for you, hopefully you'll feel a bit better each step up until you either hit "enough" or "too much" (i.e. you feel worse or get side effects).

Morning	Night	
½ (=2.5mg)	½	for 3 or more days, then
1 (=5mg)	1	for 3 or more days, then
1 ½ (=7.5mg)	1 ½	for 3 or more days, then
2 (=10mg)	2	for 3 or more days.

If not helping by here → stop taking.

Discuss with a doctor before going past this dose, but I have had rare patients on as high at 15mg twice a day to properly get things under control.

Ivabradine (Coralan):

How it works: By very specifically slowing the natural pacemaker in the heart without affecting blood pressure. A lot of people with Dysautonomia feel better (especially the hyperadrenergic variant) when the heart is regulated down to a more normal rate.

Advantages: Very targeted to reducing heart rate so a very low rate of side effects. No impact on blood pressure. No potential to interact with ADHD medications.

Disadvantages: Cost — significant more expensive that beta-blockers. Not well studied in pregnancy.

Dosage forms: 5mg (scored for ease in halving) or 7.5mg tablets

Usual side effects: The most common side effect is visual changes (usually "Lights seem very bright and there are comet tails on lights"). Stop if this occurs. Once the visual changes have resolved, and if you found a lower dose beneficial, then go back to the highest dose that didn't give side effects.

How to take: Start with ½ a 5mg tablet twice a day. Increase every 3 days until finding the right dose for you, hopefully you'll feel a bit better each step up until you either hit "enough" or "too much" (i.e. you feel worse or get side effects).

Morning	Night	
½ (=2.5mg)	½	for 3 or more days, then
1 (=5mg)	1	for 3 or more days, then
1 ½ (=7.5mg)	1 ½	for 3 or more days, then
2 (=10mg)	2	for 3 or more days.

If not helping by here → stop taking.

Discuss with a doctor before going past this dose, but I have had rare patients on as high at 22.5mg twice a day to properly get things under control.

Not recommended in pregnancy or if trying to become pregnant.

Advanced note: Whilst normally there is very little point taking both a beta-blocker and ivabradine as they both work to slow the heart, I have tried it a couple of times where the overall approach was successful but each agent alone was dose limited by side effects before an adequate benefit was achieved and so a combination of two agents, each at a low dose but working together, was required to get the job done.

Digoxin (Sigmaxin or Lanoxin):

Rationale for use: A very old medication, normally used in atrial fibrillation or heart failure, there is only one published paper of its use in POTS and that study wasn't designed to assess subjective outcomes, but rather to see how tilt table tests changed with various medications — but it showed a strong difference. In desperation, I trialled it a few years ago when there were other more conventional medication shortages (thanks COVID) and with extensive explanation that whilst it's a medication every doctor is familiar with it, it is not one with a strong evidence base. After almost 3 years, my experience has been that it does nothing for some people and is "the one" for others, with (as you'd expect) some in between. Given we're trying it only when all the standard therapies have been inadequate, this is quite impressive.

I haven't been able to determine any predictive factors of who it is more or less likely to benefit, so I have added it to the bottom of this list of things to try and see.

Dosage forms: 62.5mcg or 250mcg tablets

How to use: Unless there are concerns about severe renal failure (almost never the case in this population group), start at 62.5mcg (very low, but people are often very concerned about side effects and are more comfortable starting here) daily for a week, and then increase to 125mcg daily for a week and then check the digoxin level by a special blood test. The target blood level range seems to be the same as for other uses (as you'd expect as the point of doing levels is to avoid toxicity — usually nausea and loss of appetite).

Check the blood level **before** taking the medication after a week on 125mcg. If the

- Level is low and no change to symptoms yet — not enough → Increase the dose and recheck the level in a week
- Level is good and no change in symptoms → Not the one for you. Stop and try something else.
- Level is good and feel better → Great, take the win and stay on the dose that is helping.

- Level is low and feel better → Take the win and there's room to try more and see if it helps more.

This can be ceased suddenly without needing to be weaned off, though it will take about 5–7 days to completely wear off.

This medication crosses the placenta and has been used for treating both foetal and maternal conditions without report of foetal harm. As such, there is no contraindication for using digoxin during pregnancy or during lactation.

Coming off these regular medications:

Many patients ask, "Will I need these medications indefinitely?" Fortunately, the answer is almost always no, whether due to improvement from the exercise program or spontaneous improvement over time.

Consider attempting to reduce medications when:

1. You've achieved an optimal combination of regular therapies
2. You've been feeling well for some months

To reduce medications:

1. Attempt to wean off one medication at a time.
2. Follow the reverse of the initial "weaning up" protocol.
3. If successful, maintain the lower dose.
4. If unsuccessful, return to the lowest effective dose(s) and try again in a few months.

A typical scenario might look like this: "I was feeling pretty good on three tablets of fludrocortisone a day, so I tried gradually reducing by half a tablet each week. The first drop went fine, the second one was okay too, but when I tried going down to one and a half tablets a day, the symptoms returned. So, I went back to two tablets daily, which turned out to be the right amount for me at the time."

If you're on multiple medications:

1. Wean to the lowest effective dose of one medication.
2. Then attempt to reduce another using the same approach.

This method allows you to find the minimum effective doses across all your medications as your situation improves.

As required medications:

These agents have a relatively short duration of effect in the body so can be taken only when needed (e.g. about to do housework or exercise), but some people find they like feeling well so take them regularly through the day, which is also fine.

Pyridostigmine (Mestinon):

How it works: By inhibiting the breakdown of acetylcholine which is a major chemical messenger in the autonomic nervous system — thus magnifying various effects which helps in a large proportion of Dysautonomia cases (or as you'll see it written online sometimes "Boosts the Vagus nerve").

Dosage forms: 10mg tablets (immediate release), 60mg tablets (immediate release, can be halved), 180mg (slow release providing an effect over 12 hours, can be halved).

How to use: The effects usually last for about 4 hours but can vary a bit. So, most people take it when they get up (e.g. 7am) find that they need to take another dose again around 11am, then again mid-afternoon and may or may not take it again of an evening at their discretion. There isn't much point taking it just before bed as you'll be lying down and sleeping then anyway.

Generally, if it's working people report having energy and/or feeling better about 20 minutes after taking it and having that feeling wear off about 4 hours later, so they take it again.

Start with 10mg tablets every 4 hours as required (e.g. 7am, 11am, 3pm) during awake hours.

Increase in 10mg steps every 3 days until finding the right dose for you.

For example: Start with 10mg each dose and see how you feel. If that's okay but you think a higher dose might help more, try 20mg every 4 hours during the day for a few days. If there is no effect, or it helps a bit and you wonder if 30mg would be better, try that for a few days — and so on.

See what works best — keep increasing the dose until either there is sufficient benefit or side effects. For most people the best dose seems to be between 20mg and 60mg at a time, but I've had a few people as high as 180mg a dose and a few where 10mg each time was entirely sufficient.

If you find a dosing pattern that you feel great with — then continue at that dose

You may find that you get to the point of being able to have a different dose each time depending on how you feel or what you're doing.

Common mistakes to avoid:

1. Settling for a "good" dose (e.g. 20mg) without trying a higher dose (e.g. 30mg or more) that might be even better.

2. Giving up in the 40–60mg per dose range if there's no effect. Some people need higher doses. If you do reach the 90–120mg per dose range with no effect or side effects, that'd be quite unusual and probably worth discussing with your doctor specifically.

Usual side effects to watch out for: abdominal discomfort or cramps, excess saliva or bowel frequency. If any of these occurs then it'll only be for about 4 hours, but it's also the only way to be sure you've really given it the best go to find what's best for you. Once that or any other intolerable side effect occurs, then go back to whatever was the most helpful dose. If that dose was zero (i.e. you had side effects before benefit) then this isn't the one for you.

Midodrine (Vasodrine):

How it works: tells blood vessels to constrict.

Dosage forms: 2.5mg, 5mg and 10mg tablets. All can be halved.

Usual side effects: hairs standing on end and/or scalp and neck tingling. Rarely headache.

How to use: The effects usually last for about 3 and a half hours but can vary. Many people will leave it by the bedside, roll over and take it with a glass of water on waking, wait 15 minutes or so for it to take effect and then go about their day, taking top up doses as required.

Generally, if it is working people report having more energy or feeling better about 15–20 minutes after taking it and having that feeling wear off about 3–3 1/2 hours later — so they take it again. Sometimes a half dose will be enough for follow-up doses in a day.

I generally recommend starting at 2.5mg/dose for a few days and working up from there as tolerated and required. For some people a low dose is enough a couple of times a day, or just if required before they exercise or have to be upright for a period. I also have a couple of severely afflicted patients we have slowly and carefully worked up as high as 15mg up to 4 times a day. Everyone is different.

<u>Important note</u>: It comes with a warning not to lie down for some hours after taking. That's really for people with Parkinson's disease where people can have very (very) high blood pressure when lying flat. This is not really an issue in the general patient population discussed here, and most people don't take it if they're going to be lying around anyway.

Considerations for Existing Medications

Many people with Dysautonomia are already taking some medications for other reasons when diagnosed. A particularly relevant example is the **Oral Contraceptive Pill (OCP)**.

Most menstruating patients report their Dysautonomia symptoms worsen significantly just before and during their period. Continuous use of the OCP (skipping the sugar/placebo pills) can often help manage this pattern. This approach:

- Is safe for long-term use,
- Does not affect future fertility,
- Can help manage iron deficiency if that's a factor, and
- May help stabilise symptoms throughout the month.

However, some people may experience side effects or have other considerations that make the OCP unsuitable. These issues are best discussed with your regular medical practitioner.

The section on associated conditions later in this guide covers many other medications you might be taking. The most important thing is to keep your healthcare providers informed about all your medications so they can adjust your treatment plan accordingly.

Things to consider avoiding if possible:

Anything that increases noradrenaline (also called norepinephrine in North America) levels can be problematic so it's generally advised to avoid medications known as SNRIs (serotonin noradrenaline reuptake inhibitors) such as bupropion (Wellbutrin, Zyban or Contrave), venlafaxine or desvenlafaxine (Efexor/Effexor depending on the country, or Pristiq), or duloxetine (Cymbalta).

A good proportion of people do seem to tolerate them without issue (everyone is different), particularly duloxetine. If there is a compelling reason to want to try and no other alternatives, it is reasonable to start with a low dose and see what happens after discussing with your individual practitioner. Sometimes it just means a larger dose of something else will be required to offset it.

Similarly, some ADHD medications work by increasing adrenaline release in the brain, so having something that has the opposite effect doesn't seem wise. This can usually be worked around by picking agents that don't penetrate the blood-brain barrier (i.e. avoid propranolol). My general impression has been that lisdexamfetamine (Vyvanse) isn't an issue for most people, whilst several people have issues with atomoxetine (Strattera), and methylphenidate (Concerta) falls somewhere in between.

Less well-established agents:

Naltrexone:

This was adopted out of the chronic fatigue syndrome literature and does help a good proportion of people a bit, but rarely lifechanging in my experience (despite the many anecdotes online).

It is one of the antidotes for opioids (morphine, oxycodone, fentanyl and related compounds) but in this protocol it is started at such tiny doses that you'd think wouldn't have much of an effect, but which over time can help modulate body chemistry in beneficial ways. It doesn't work though if you're also taking opioids regularly[19].

Dosage forms: As it's in such low doses it will need to be compounded by a specialist pharmacy. Get quotes from several compounding pharmacies as prices can vary considerably.

How to use it: There are many different protocols and the one I was taught and have generally used is[20]:

- Start at 0.5mg or 1mg each morning for 2 weeks, then
- Increase in 0.5mg steps every fortnight (1mg each morning for 2 weeks, then 1.5mg daily for a fortnight, then 2mg a day, and so on) until finding the best dose.
- If you get to 3mg a day with no improvement — just give up. It's alright to stop suddenly at such low doses.

- Otherwise, if you think it is helping, just increase every fortnight as long as stepping it up helps. At some point (usually around the 3.5–5mg range) people will increase the dose and feel worse — at which point go back to the "best dose" and stick with that. I've had 120kg+ patients feel best on as low as 1.5mg/day and other people who got to doses as high as 9mg/day — but both are quite unusual.

---

[19] These medications have many different brand names across different countries — your pharmacist or doctor can help identify specific products if needed.
[20] This is significantly slower than the standard fibromyalgia treatment protocol.

- It's often worth getting prescriptions for a couple of different strengths to streamline dosing and to reduce the need to refill prescriptions. I usually give prescriptions for 0.5mg and 1.5mg capsules and allow the patient to combine them as required to get the protocol dose each week until they find the most effective dose for them.

The most common side effects are insomnia or vivid dreams. These often settle after a few weeks or can be minimised by taking it in the morning.

SSRIs (Selective Serotonin Reuptake Inhibitors):

Unlike SNRIs, which can worsen symptoms, SSRIs are generally well-tolerated in POTS patients and have often been started before the diagnosis is made — remember the bit about people commonly being diagnosed with anxiety or depression?

Common SSRIs like sertraline (Zoloft), escitalopram (Lexapro), or fluoxetine (Prozac) may even help some patients feel a bit better. Whether this is via a direct effect on the condition or by helping with associated anxiety or depression, either from the condition itself or the impact on quality of life[21] in many ways doesn't matter and probably varies from individual to individual. Some people may experience no benefit, while others might find significant relief.

If you're already on an SSRI, there's usually no need to stop it unless it seems to be causing problems. If you're considering starting or stopping an SSRI, always discuss this with your healthcare provider. Never stop these medications suddenly as this can cause withdrawal symptoms and potentially worsen both mood and Dysautonomia symptoms.

Clonidine:

A centrally acting (at the level of the brain) anti-sympathetic nervous system agent.

---

[21] Rarely, if ever, is a life afflicted by Dysautonomia the one people were hoping to have.

Generally recommended in hyperadrenergic POTS or in the very rare situation when the blood pressure rises dramatically on standing.

I only trial this rarely as I find it makes people too sleepy even when given at night. I generally trial it only when everything else has failed though so I am using it only in the most severe cases. Some colleagues who use it earlier in their algorithms report different results.

Desmopressin:

A synthetic version of the hormone vasopressin, also known as anti-diuretic hormone. Works by telling the kidneys to retain water and causing vasoconstriction (blood vessels to squeeze) — which sounds fabulous and exactly what is needed, so why not start with this?

Unfortunately, it retains water — but not salt, so there is a risk of diluting yourself (hyponatremia) which, as the sodium concentration in the body gets lower, will first cause confusion, then seizures and potentially, if it gets low enough, death. As long as it's carefully monitored and the patient and those around them know to stop if any hint of confusion occurs then it is reasonable to trial, but it is relatively difficult to monitor, and I've only had two Dysautonomia patients stick with it for any reasonable amount of time.

The best niche is probably to just take it at night to decrease overnight urination if that is an issue.

Talking to Your Doctor About Dysautonomia Management

So, you've read through this guide and you're thinking, "Hey, this sounds great, but it's very different from the approach my doctor is taking. How do I bring any of this up without sounding like I'm challenging my doctor?"

The reality is your practitioner probably isn't a specialist in this emerging and complex area and would love to know more, so if approached in a sense of collaboration they will likely appreciate some help in helping you, if so done politely and with respect for their likely very limited time.

Before Your Appointment

1. **Do Your Homework**: Jot down the main points you want to discuss. Maybe it's a new medication, or a different approach to exercise. Whatever it is, have it clear in your mind.

2. **Bring Backup**: Take a copy of this guide with you, or at least the relevant sections (it's why there's a variety of printable summaries at the back which are also available online[22]). Highlight the parts you want to talk about. It's not about proving you're right, it's about starting a conversation.

3. **Write Down Your Questions**: Trust me, you'll forget half of them once you're in the doctor's office, and half of the answers as you walk out the door (it's been formally studied). It's not you, it's just how our brains work.

During Your Appointment

1. **Start on a Positive Note**: Your doctor is there to help, they're on your side and want to help you. Try something like, "Dr. Stethoscope, I really appreciate the care you've been giving me. I've been doing some research to better

---

[22] http://aionhealth.com.au/Dysautonomia-Resources/

understand my condition, and I'd love to get your thoughts on a few things."

2. **Be Clear and Specific**: Don't beat around the bush. Say something like, "I've been reading this guide on Dysautonomia management, and it mentions using fludrocortisone differently than we've been doing. Could we talk about that?"

3. **Ask, Don't Demand**: It's a team effort, and your doctor has years or decades of training and experience. Ask questions like, "What do you think about this approach?" or "Have you tried this with other patients?"

4. **Listen**: Your doctor might have some really good reasons for doing things differently. They may need to work within local healthcare system constraints, like insurance requirements or medication availability in your area. Or maybe there's something specific about your case that makes it unsuitable. Be open to their perspective.

5. **Suggest a Trial**: If you're both open to it, you could say something like, "Would it be worth trying this for a month to see if it helps?"

6. **Write it down**: Whatever plan you agree on moving forward, write it down before you leave the room so you know what it is and can more easily share it with anyone supporting you.

After Your Appointment

1. **Follow Up**: If you decide to try something new, make sure to schedule a follow-up appointment to discuss how it's going.

2. **Be Patient**: Remember how I said earlier that everyone with Dysautonomia is different? Well, that means finding the right treatment can take time. Don't get discouraged if the first thing you try doesn't work perfectly.

3. **Consider a Second Opinion**: If you feel like you're not being heard, or if you and your doctor just can't seem to

get on the same page, it's okay to seek a second opinion. It's not about replacing your doctor, it's about getting the best care possible.

A Word on "Doctor Shopping"

It's important to distinguish between seeking a second opinion and what's often termed "Doctor Shopping". Seeking a second opinion is a valid and often recommended practice, especially when dealing with complex conditions like Dysautonomia. It involves consulting another qualified healthcare professional to get an additional perspective on your diagnosis or treatment plan.

This is distinct from the practice of going from doctor to doctor until you find one who tells you what you want to hear — this is **not** a good idea, potentially leading to inconsistent care, missed diagnoses, or inappropriate treatments. It's about finding a doctor who listens to you, explains things clearly, and works with you to find the best treatment plan — not a rubber stamp. You're the person suffering, and shouldn't have to be the doctor too — don't try to be.

Remember, the goal here is to work together with your healthcare team, and Effective Dysautonomia management often requires a long-term relationship with your healthcare provider, allowing them to understand the nuances of your condition over time. You're bringing valuable information about your experiences and what you've learned, and they're bringing their medical expertise. Together, you can hopefully find the best way to manage your unique situation.

If your doctor is interested in learning more, feel free to share this guide with them — it's what it's for. The more healthcare providers who understand Dysautonomia, the better it is for all of us.

Special circumstances

Most Dysautonomia suffers feel worse with:

- Hotter weather (and better when its cooler. Unfortunately, it's difficult to live in a walk-in freezer or to move to Iceland).
- Just before their period (see Oral Contraceptive Pill as mentioned earlier).
- After an acute infection (especially Epstein-Barr Virus, Influenza or Covid).

At these times (or with any other cause of a flare in symptoms) they may need higher dosing than they usually do for a while. For most people that will take the form of either working up the fludrocortisone for a bit, or taking more of the as required medications.

There's a more detailed section on a variety of special situations later after Associated Conditions and before the Conclusion and Extra Resources.

Alternative Therapies for Dysautonomia

Understandably, a lot of my patients have tried a remarkably wide range of alternative therapies — starting with various supplements[23], through to faith-based and increasingly exotic (and expensive) laser and "energy-based" treatments. While I acknowledge I might just be seeing the group where these didn't help, it's noteworthy that despite sometimes spending astonishing sums of money — and occasionally suffering significant injuries — these patients still ended up seeing me.

Conventional medical treatments are exactly that for a simple reason — they reliably work. That's how treatments become 'conventional' — by proving themselves effective in properly conducted studies and then in real-world clinical practice, not through marketing campaigns or testimonials. When alternative treatments are properly studied and proven to work, they become conventional medicine — they stop being 'alternative'. The fact that most alternative treatments remain 'alternative' tells you something important: they either haven't been properly tested, failed when tested (though you won't hear about these negative studies from people trying to sell them), or worse, keep being promoted despite being proven ineffective[24].

I'll use whatever works — as long as it's safe when used properly, and actually helps a worthwhile proportion of patients. If you choose to explore less well-established treatment options, it's important to approach these with a critical, sceptical eye and always discuss them with your healthcare provider.

---

[23] To the point where I can recognise which naturopath they've seen by their supplement cocktail. Interestingly, each naturopath seems to have their own standard 'fatigue protocol' that they recommend regardless of cause — rather undermining any claims of providing highly individualised therapy.

[24] A special note on 'quantum' claims: While quantum mechanics is a fascinating field of physics dealing with atomic-scale phenomena, the term is frequently misused in alternative medicine marketing. If someone promotes a treatment using quantum terminology but can't explain how it works in regular medical terms, they're almost certainly using scientific-sounding words to mask a lack of evidence. The same goes for vague claims about 'vibrations,' 'energy fields,' or 'resonance.' Save your time and money for something that may actually work.

Important Considerations

- **Safety First**: Always consult your healthcare provider before starting any alternative therapy.

- **Evidence-Based Approach**: Look for therapies with some scientific backing.

- **Complementary, Not Replacement**: If you do want to explore them, alternative therapies should complement, not replace, conventional treatments.

- **Individual Responses Vary**: What works for one person may not work for another.

- **Cost-Benefit Analysis**: Consider the financial cost against potential benefits.

- **Potential Interactions**: Some alternative therapies can interact with conventional medications. This is why it is important to let your healthcare providers know if you are planning to trial an alternative therapy, even if it seems harmless.

Essentially this guide includes a wide variety of treatments that my patients and I have found to <u>actually work</u>, be safe, and be affordable — I suggest trying these proven approaches before investing time and money elsewhere.

Emerging Treatments

These are interventions where there is currently insufficient high-quality evidence to make a recommendation, with more research and clinical trials needed to establish efficacy, but that people are watching hopefully. This is a summary of my current understanding of various treatments under investigation at the moment — some are more promising or further along than others.

Cutaneous Vagal nerve stimulation (cVNS or tVNS): Cutaneous vagal nerve stimulation has gained interest as a non-invasive approach for managing Dysautonomia in recent years. The vagus nerve is a very large nerve which extends from the brain to monitor and control the internal organs from jaw to the navel, including importantly the heart, gut, and blood vessels. The only place it connects to the surface is a small branch to the outer ear and some skin around that area (specifically the lump of cartilage at the front of the ear canal — known as the tragus).

The theory is that by targeting this branch with electrical pulsations, the vagus nerve can be stimulated to modulate autonomic nervous system activity, particularly enhancing parasympathetic tone and reducing sympathetic overactivity (which are often dysregulated in Dysautonomia) with hopefully the result of feeling better.

Initial pilot studies have demonstrated that cVNS may improve symptoms in patients with POTS and Long COVID by stabilising heart rate and blood pressure responses during orthostatic stress. Preliminary findings suggest potential benefits, but larger, randomised controlled trials are needed to confirm efficacy. I've had a few patients try it so far, and whilst it does seem to change their pulse rate, their overall wellbeing and function didn't seem to change markedly.

The exact protocol of the best intensity, the best frequency of stimulation and how long/how often to use it remains to be established.

cVNS is generally well-tolerated, with most adverse events being mild and transient, such as local skin irritation at the site of stimulation. Rarely, patients may experience headaches or dizziness, which are typically self-limiting. Long-term safety data is still limited, particularly regarding frequent use over an extended period.

One issue likely to confound things is the variability of Dysautonomia patients. Different types, from different causes, in different individuals, makes it hard to believe there will be a single approach or protocol that will prove beneficial for most people. If it is shown to be effective the difficulty will be in knowing who is best to use it on. It may be another case of trying and seeing what happens.

Currently, if you do wish to try it, the research suggests trying a (relatively cheap preferably — the price can vary a lot online) TENS device (transcutaneous electrical nerve stimulation) with an ear clip on the tragus, at a frequency of 10 Hertz (Hz) (this is one of the main things yet to be determined), turned up to a level where you can feel it, but not so much that it is painful, for 30–90 minutes a day, most days of the week, for 4 to 8 weeks. If it seems to be helping → Great! Keep it going. If you don't seem to be improving, then maybe give it a miss and focus on other therapies.

Endothelial dysfunction treatments: There is evidence demonstrating endothelial dysfunction (where the layer of cells lining the blood vessels does not function properly) in patients with POTS. What has yet to occur is a study demonstrating evidence of benefit in trying to improve this.

Hydroxyethylrutoside (Oxerutins, Paroven, Venoruton): Available on pharmacy shelves in Australia, online as a supplement in the USA and Canada, but requiring a prescription in some of Europe. This medication has long been used to treat chronic venous incompetence, where it helps improve blood flow and reduce swelling in legs with poor circulation. Given the similarity between these symptoms and the venous pooling seen in some Dysautonomia patients, I innovated by trying this medication in cases where patients had significant venous pooling (purple blotchy congested legs, or pelvic congestion) and were not responding well to, or were unsuitable for, the standard therapy of compression garments. After explaining the lack of experience with it in this patient population and explaining the rationale, I suggested that people try it, given its established safety profile and relatively low cost. Standard dosing is 60mg twice a day, though I've had a couple of people report benefit from higher doses. So far, all patients I've prescribed it to have reported benefit — though it's still a small number of cases. I usually suggest people buy a bottle and if it helps great, if not — don't buy another bottle.

Hyperbaric Oxygen Therapy (HBOT): Hyperbaric oxygen therapy (HBOT) has emerged as a promising treatment option, particularly in Long COVID cases where it has shown significant improvements in cognitive function, fatigue, and quality of life in several controlled trials[25,26]. HBOT involves breathing 100% oxygen in a pressurised chamber, typically at 2–2.4 times normal atmospheric pressure for 90 minute sessions. While the exact mechanisms aren't fully understood, the treatment may work by improving tissue oxygenation, reducing inflammation, and supporting cellular repair processes. Results in Long COVID patients have been encouraging, with benefits persisting even a year after treatment in some studies. However, there is not yet evidence for its effectiveness in other forms of Dysautonomia.

Importantly, "hyperbaric" treatments offered by some alternative practitioners using soft chambers at lower pressures have not demonstrated the same benefits — the studied effects specifically require medical-grade chambers capable of reaching at least twice normal atmospheric pressure. The treatment requires specialised hospital or medical facilities and can be costly, with a typical session costing several hundred dollars. Given the limited availability of proper hyperbaric chambers and significant cost (several hundred dollars per session currently locally), this remains an investigational approach. While published protocols

[25] Katz AA, Wainwright S, Kelly MP, Albert P and Byrne R (2024) Hyperbaric oxygen effectively addresses the pathophysiology of long COVID: clinical review. Front. Med. 11:1354088. doi: 10.3389/fmed.2024.1354088
[26] Hadanny, A., Zilberman-Itskovich, S., Catalogna, M. et al. Long term outcomes of hyperbaric oxygen therapy in post covid condition: longitudinal follow-up of a randomized controlled trial. Sci Rep 14, 3604 (2024). https://doi.org/10.1038/s41598-024-53091-3

often describe 40 sessions over 2 months, my clinical experience to date suggests that if HBOT is going to help, improvements are often seen with far fewer sessions. If no benefit is observed after 5–6 sessions, it's probably reasonable to discontinue treatment. On the other hand, if you're feeling significantly better or even 'cured' at some point (maybe as few as 8–10 treatments), it would seem reasonable to discuss this with your hyperbaric specialist — they may recommend stopping or a few additional sessions to consolidate the improvement, with the option to return for further 'top-up' treatments if needed in the future[27]. As the optimal treatment protocol is still being determined, it's best to be guided by the hyperbaric specialist facilitating your treatment. However, more research is needed before HBOT can be recommended as a standard treatment option.

Intravenous Immunoglobulin (IVIG): Derived from blood donors this is relatively difficult to get and whilst generally well-tolerated does carry some risks (including fever, headache, flushing and generally feeling "Blah" for a bit), particularly when first starting. That said there is a very promising though also very small retrospective analysis[28] of 38 patients that found IVIG was effective and safe in a subset of patients with autoimmune Dysautonomias, including postural tachycardia syndrome (POTS) and gastrointestinal dysmotility. 83.5% of patients improved on IVIG, with a mean pre-treatment functional ability score of 21% (mostly bedridden) improving to 74% (nearing able to return to work/school) after at least 1 year of IVIG.

A more recent follow-up randomised controlled trial[29] (the gold standard for testing treatments, where participants were randomly assigned to receive either IVIG or a comparison treatment) of 30

---

[27] Given the highly limited availability, it's in no one's interest to do anything more than the minimum number of required sessions. Better to free up the spot and help someone else.

[28] Schofield JR, Chemali KR. Intravenous Immunoglobulin Therapy in Refractory Autoimmune Dysautonomias: A Retrospective Analysis of 38 Patients. Am J Ther. 2019 Sep/Oct;26(5):570-582. doi: 10.1097/MJT.0000000000000778. PMID: 29781817.

[29] Vernino S, Hopkins S, Bryarly M, Hernandez RS, Salter A. Randomized controlled trial of intravenous immunoglobulin for autoimmune postural orthostatic tachycardia syndrome (iSTAND). Clin Auton Res. 2024 Feb;34(1):153-163. doi: 10.1007/s10286-024-01020-9. Epub 2024 Feb 4. PMID: 38311655.

POTS patients compared IVIG to albumin infusions over 12 weeks. While IVIG showed a slightly higher response rate (47% versus 39%), this wasn't statistically significant. Both groups improved somewhat, possibly just from the volume expansion effects. While this study doesn't support IVIG as being clearly effective, it was a small relatively short trial and demonstrates that more research is needed.

Microbiome analysis: Still very much a work in progress. The gut bacteria of individuals with POTS are often different to health controls, but unfortunately our ability to meaningfully manipulate that flora in a useful way is still lacking, no matter what your local naturopath or someone online might be trying to sell you. I've seen a lot of people spend a lot of money on this approach and yet they were still seeing me.

Stellate Ganglion Block (SGB): Involves injecting local anaesthetic around a collection of sympathetic nerves in the neck called the stellate ganglion. While traditionally used to treat chronic pain conditions, there is growing interest in its potential role in managing Dysautonomia, particularly in cases involving heightened sympathetic nervous system activity (hyperadrenergic POTS) or as part of Long COVID. The procedure temporarily blocks signals through these nerves, potentially "resetting" the autonomic nervous system. Early case reports and small studies have shown promising results in some patients, with improvements in heart rate, blood pressure regulation, and quality of life, though larger controlled trials are still needed to confirm these benefits.

The procedure is relatively quick (usually under 30 minutes) and is performed by pain specialists or radiologist using imaging guidance. While generally considered safe, potential side effects include temporary hoarseness and a drooping eyelid. More serious complications, while rare, are possible any time needles are placed deep in the neck. The duration of benefit varies significantly — some patients report improvements lasting months, while others see little or no benefit. Given the invasive nature, significant cost (often several hundred or thousands of dollars per procedure), and limited evidence base, SGB is typically considered only after more established treatments have been tried. Additionally, you may need repeated treatments to maintain any benefits, making this a potentially expensive option with no guarantee of success.

Red Light Therapy: Also known as photobiomodulation, this treatment involves exposure to specific wavelengths of red and near-infrared light, typically via LED panels or laser devices. While heavily marketed online and through some clinics, evidence for its effectiveness in Dysautonomia is extremely limited. A few small studies suggest modest improvements in fatigue in other conditions, but these results haven't yet been reliably demonstrated in Dysautonomia patients. Claims about its effects on brain function particularly strain credibility — skulls being remarkably good at protecting the brain by blocking things from getting through — including light. While generally safe if proper eye protection is used, the significant cost of treatment or home devices may not be justified given the current lack of evidence. As with many emerging treatments, be wary of marketing claims that exceed the available scientific evidence.

Transcranial Direct Current Stimulation (tDCS): Non-invasive brain stimulation technique using weak electrical currents to the scalp, theoretically modulating brain activity. This is not something I claim any expertise with, but some small early studies suggest it may help with the brain fog associated with Dysautonomia and Long COVID. The optimal treatment protocols (current strength, duration, electrode placement) aren't established, and results have been inconsistent. While generally safe when properly administered in clinical settings, home devices marketed online should be approached with caution — they often lack proper safety controls and haven't been validated for treating Dysautonomia. Save your money until we have better evidence.

Very Low-Dose Naltrexone (VLDN) and Alternative Protocols: While the standard LDN protocol was discussed earlier, some practitioners promote various alternative approaches, including ultra-low doses (under 0.1mg) or variable dosing schedules. Despite some enthusiastic anecdotal reports, proper studies validating these modifications are currently lacking. Given the time and expense involved in extended dose experimentation, at this stage, I generally suggest moving on to something else rather than spending months trialling different doses indefinitely.

Considering Emerging Treatments — A Practical Approach:

When deciding which emerging treatments to discuss with your healthcare team, consider these factors:

1. Likelihood of Benefit

- How proportion of people seem to respond? (e.g. the initial IVIG study suggested improvement in about 80% of patients vs. cVNS which seems to help a smaller percentage)
- How significant is the improvement when it works? (e.g. IVIG can be life-changing for some, while red light therapy seems to offer modest benefits at best)
- How long do benefits typically last? (e.g. SGBs may need repeated treatments every few months vs. HBOT where benefits have lasted a year or more by some studies)
- How consistent are the benefits? (e.g. a treatment that helps 80% of people get somewhat better might be worth trying before one that dramatically helps 20% but does nothing for the rest)

2. Safety and Risk

- How invasive is the treatment?
- What are the potential side effects?
- Is it reversible?

3. Evidence Quality

- Are there controlled studies or just case reports?
- How many people have been studied?
- Did they look to see if the benefits lasted?

- Did the people selling it produce the evidence?

4. Cost and Accessibility

- What are the total costs involved?
  - Is it covered by insurance?
- Is it available in your area?
- How many sessions/treatments are needed?

5. Place in therapy

- Could it be useful as a "rescue" treatment even if not practical for everyday use? (e.g. IV saline or SGB might be worth considering for managing severe flares or special occasions, even if they're not suitable for regular use)

6. Current Treatment Status

- Have you tried all standard treatments first?
- Could this complement your current treatments?
- Would it require stopping any current treatments?

Generally, it makes sense to prioritise treatments that are less invasive, better studied, more affordable, and more accessible for regular use. For example, trying cVNS with a relatively inexpensive TENS unit might be worth discussing before considering more invasive or expensive options like HBOT or IVIG. However, it's also worth knowing about more intensive options that might be helpful during severe flares, even if they're not practical for everyday use.

Remember that what works best for one person may not work for another — this is particularly true with emerging treatments where we're still learning who might benefit most.

Cautions

- Beware of sensationalised headlines; always read the full article.
- Be sceptical of "miracle cures" or treatments that seem too good to be true. Just because people say it's good doesn't mean it is — especially if they're selling it.
- Remember that what seems to work in early studies often doesn't pan out in the real world or for everyone (disappointingly). I've seen a lot of early promising work fail to live up to the hype and hope over the decades.

Staying informed about Dysautonomia research can be empowering, but it's important to approach new information critically and always discuss significant findings with your healthcare team before making treatment decisions — especially if there are potential risks to your health or wallet.

Associated Conditions

Key Points

Common co-existing conditions:

- Mast Cell Activation Syndrome,
- Hypermobility,
- ADHD,
- Autism Spectrum Disorder,
- Migraines, and
- Endometriosis.

Management implications:

- Treatment interactions.
- Medication choices.
- Exercise modifications.
- Specialist involvement.

Approach:

- Manage all conditions when possible.
- Monitor interactions.
- Regular review.
- Adjust as needed.

Dysautonomia, and particularly POTS, often occurs alongside other health conditions. If you think you might have one of these conditions, raise your concerns with your regular doctor.

Some of the more common and important conditions are:

Mast Cell Activation Syndrome (MCAS, "Em-Cas"):

MCAS happens when certain cells in your immune system — called mast cells — become overactive. Think of mast cells as your body's security guards. Usually, they help protect you from threats, but in MCAS, they start overreacting to things they shouldn't. The MCAS diagnosis fills an important gap, describing reactions more severe than atopy (a tendency toward allergic responses like rashes and hay fever) but not as severe as anaphylaxis (life-threatening allergic reactions).

First proposed in 2010, it's a fairly new diagnosis which many medical practitioners are still learning about. While it has become very popular in alternative medicine circles — risking being diagnosed when other conditions are actually responsible for the presentation — MCAS is essentially an umbrella term that describes a clinical presentation rather than a specific diagnosis. It involves inappropriate mast cell activation, leading to symptoms such as allergic reactions and gastrointestinal issues. In 2022 an expert working group expanded the definition of MCAS to include both primary and secondary mast cell disorders.

To be formally diagnosed with MCAS currently[30], you need:

- Clear physical signs of reactions involving at least two body systems (like skin rashes plus breathing problems, or stomach issues plus heart symptoms) — just feeling tired or foggy-headed alone isn't enough,

---

[30] Currently the complete technical diagnostic criteria for MCAS are:
1. Episodic, objective signs and symptoms consistent with mast cell activation involving at least two of the following organ systems: skin, upper or lower respiratory systems, gastrointestinal, or cardiovascular. Note that subjective symptoms alone (fatigue, difficulty concentrating) in the absence of signs and symptoms in two other organ systems specified above does **not** warrant an evaluation for mast cell disorders.
2. Evidence of systemic mast cell-mediator release, corresponding temporally to the presence of symptoms. In case of frequent recurrent episodes, mediator release should be ideally documented on at least two occasions. Serum total tryptase is the most specific for mast cell activation, and an increase from the patient's baseline to a level of (1.2 x baseline) + 2 ng/mL is considered indicative of mast cell activation.
3. Response to medications that stabilise mast cells, reduce mast cell mediator production, block mediator release, or inhibit the actions of mediators.

- Blood or urine tests showing that mast cells are overactive during these reactions (proof that the symptoms are actually coming from mast cells), and
- Improvement when taking medications that calm down mast cells.

While meeting all the detailed criteria may be important for insurance or governmental purposes, capturing the required blood test evidence of mast cell overactivation can be notoriously difficult. So just as I don't tell the person with a good story of Dysautonomia and a postural tachycardia of only +27 bpm, instead of the official ≥30 bpm, I personally don't insist on capturing these hard-to-get test results unless they're needed for official documentation

Instead, if someone reports likely mast cell mediated symptoms — such as developing lots of food sensitivities, gastrointestinal issues (pain, heartburn, nausea, vomiting, diarrhoea), skin problems (rashes, flushing, itching), or frequent sinusitis or hay-fever symptoms — I usually skip to criteria 3 and see if a treatment trial helps. If it does, I call it an "MCAS-like" condition rather than formal MCAS, since we haven't met all the official criteria.

One thing to note: symptoms like headaches, fatigue, brain fog, and trouble concentrating can happen with MCAS, but they're also really common in Dysautonomia generally. So, I usually try getting the Dysautonomia under better control first before trialling MCAS therapies.

For the treatment trial (which I borrowed from an immunologist who specialises in this), we typically use two types of antihistamines together: a non-sedating antihistamine that blocks 'H1' receptors (the kind most people are familiar with from pharmacy shelves) along with another that blocks 'H2' receptors (these are usually used for reducing stomach acid, but in MCAS we're using them for their antihistamine effects).

Usual regimen

H1 blocker (non-sedating): In most countries these are all available over the counter at the pharmacy. The "is it MCAS-like" trial consists of twice the standard dose, twice a day of either fexofenadine, cetirizine, levocetirizine, loratadine or desloratadine. Whichever is your favourite or cheapest at the pharmacy that week. That said, some people say one is markedly better than another for them but the only way to be sure is to cycle through and find out if one works better for you than another. It won't be the case though that one works remarkably well if the others do nothing, so if the first one you try has no impact then it is unlikely another will.

H1 Blocker	Standard Dosing	MCAS-trial Dosing
Fexofenadine	180mg daily	360mg twice a day (bd)
Cetirizine	10mg daily	20mg twice a day
Levocetirizine	5mg daily	10mg twice a day
Loratadine	10mg daily	20mg twice a day
Desloratadine	5mg daily	10mg twice a day

(Pick one and try it for a week or two — if it doesn't help then stop).

PLUS a

H2 Blocker: Famotidine or Nizatidine again at high dose. In most countries these require a prescription. These are usually used to decrease stomach acidity in reflux, but have seen a lot less use in recent decades as more effective agents for this became available (proton pump inhibitors — which do NOT have any antihistamine effects), making them at times hard to get. A lot of people consider famotidine the better agent but I haven't noticed that specifically, and I suspect people just don't use "enough" nizatidine to be equivalent. Also, some people just seem to do better with one than the other, but once again if you try one and it does nothing then it is reasonable to give up as it probably isn't MCAS causing the symptoms.

H2 Blocker	Standard	MCAS-trial
Famotidine	10–20mg twice a day	40mg twice a day
Nizatidine	150mg twice a day	300mg twice a day

As this is a lot of tablets to start with (four of the regular antihistamines and two to four of the H2 blockers each day), if you do find this approach helps, it's worth trying to gradually reduce one type at a time to find the lowest doses that keep your symptoms under control.

I've seen some immunologists push dosing as high as double what I've described to try controlling symptoms. While these medications are very safe — even in Dysautonomia patients who seem prone to rare and unusual side effects — that's still a significant number of pills to take daily. In my experience, if this dosing isn't helping, it's usually better to move on and try something else rather than keep increasing things hoping for success.

If the antihistamine combination helps but doesn't completely control your symptoms, there are two main options we might try next:

- Montelukast 10mg daily (I haven't found this particularly helpful, even other doctors report better success), or
- Ketotifen, starting at 0.5mg twice daily and gradually increasing over a few weeks to 2mg twice daily if needed. This medication is particularly interesting because it both blocks histamine and helps prevent mast cells from releasing it in the first place.

Beyond that you're into territory where it's best to consult with a specialist immunologist[31].

---

[31] Though there are several other therapeutic options here — we're probably getting beyond the scope of a guide that's supposed to be about Dysautonomia.

Hypermobility:

How flexible we are is highly variable across the population, from stiff ("dances like a tin soldier") through people who are very flexible ("dances like a swan" or a born gymnast) to people so flexible it causes problems ("too floppy to dance").

Whilst in many ways an advantage, being very flexible does increase the risk of Dysautonomia. At an extreme is a genetic condition called Ehlers-Danlos Syndrome, (EDS) with up to half of people with the most common variant (hypermobile EDS — hEDS) being diagnosed with POTS as well in some series. Going the other way, at least until Long Covid, up to 31% of POTS patients meet the clinical criteria for hEDS with an additional 24% exhibiting generalised joint hypermobility without meeting the full (quite complex) hEDS criteria[32].

You don't need to meet the full criteria for EDS to have hypermobility that causes issues. Many people are hypermobile without meeting the EDS diagnostic criteria, and this 'benign joint hypermobility' can still affect how Dysautonomia presents and how it should be managed, particularly regarding exercise and physical rehabilitation approaches. The key is working with your physiotherapist or exercise physiologist to develop strategies that take your individual level of joint mobility into account, whether or not you meet formal EDS diagnostic criteria.

Presumably, the link is that the changes in the tissues that make joints stretchy also affects the blood vessels in unfortunate ways, so that there is a predisposition to ANS dysfunction. This makes it more likely that when a second factor (e.g. a virus) comes along and adds further stress, the body which coped with one issue can't cope with two.

For most people being assessed and formally diagnosed or not doesn't make a great deal of difference, as having a label or not doesn't change anything practically (unless dealing with insurers or governmental bodies).

---

[32] https://www.ehlers-danlos.com/what-is-hsd/

What hypermobility does impact is likely prognosis and the physical rehabilitation plan. Research suggests that people with more severe hypermobility typically don't respond as well to the standard exercise therapy for Dysautonomia as their stiffer peers. That doesn't mean it isn't worth doing — but if there's a choice in the limited therapy hours between maintaining musculoskeletal strength and conditioning and Dysautonomia therapy, then focus on the musculoskeletal work.

Attention-Deficit/Hyperactivity Disorder (ADHD):

A condition characterised by persistent inattention, hyperactivity, and impulsivity that can interfere with daily functioning and development. In one series 51% of individuals diagnosed with ADHD had generalised joint hypermobility. I have no idea how being extra-bendy causes brain effects.

Some studies suggest that up to 25–30 % of patients with POTS may also have ADHD, especially in adolescents and young adults. The exact prevalence varies across different studies, but the comorbidity rate is generally considered to be higher than in the general population.

Practically this can influence therapy in terms of medication choices, both in avoiding negative interactions (as covered earlier) and also in trying to minimise the frequency of medications a day (i.e. trying to keep to once or twice a day dosing instead of complex regimens if possible).

Autism Spectrum Disorder (ASD):

Even less well studied, and specific prevalence rates are not yet well established, but the research to date is clearly indicating that autonomic issues, including orthostatic intolerance, are more common in people with ASD.

Migraines:

Migraines are distinct from headaches, which are nearly universal in Dysautonomia sufferers, but which usually settle well with standard therapies as already outlined. Studies suggest that up to 40–60 % of individuals with POTS experience migraines. This is a much higher prevalence than in the general population, where migraines affect about 12% of people. Presumably this is due to a shared origin in dysfunction in the autonomic nervous system. Specifically, issues with blood vessel regulation, abnormal blood flow, and dysregulation of neurotransmitters like serotonin are implicated in both conditions.

The presence of migraines can exacerbate the symptoms of POTS and vice versa. For example, the orthostatic intolerance in POTS may trigger or worsen migraines, and the pain and discomfort of migraines can make managing POTS symptoms more difficult.

As such, quite apart from treating the misery that is a migraine, treating the migraine can be important in helping the Dysautonomia. Whilst propranolol is indicated for both conditions and so is often a good place to start, if it is not sufficiently effective or tolerated there are many other options. Unfortunately, the standard cheaper preventive treatments don't seem to be as effective or as well tolerated as in the general migraineur population. However, whilst still expensive, the newest class of preventive medications — known as CGRP (calcitonin gene-related peptide) antagonists (Aimovig, Ajovy, Emgality, Vyepti, Qulipta) — do seem both very well tolerated and quite effective.

Endometriosis:

One study reported that 20% of women with POTS reported having endometriosis, compared to only 5% in an age matched control group. This difference is statistically significant, suggesting a notable association between the two conditions.

The exact mechanisms linking POTS and endometriosis are not fully understood, though the obvious speculation is that the inflammatory processes involved in endometriosis could contribute to autonomic dysfunction. Additionally, both conditions may share common risk factors, such as hormonal changes and immune system disorders, so once again treating one may help the other, but this is not yet established.

On the other hand, they're both miserable conditions so it makes sense to treat both even if a treatment for one won't reliably help the other.

Small Fibre Neuropathy:

Small fibre neuropathy, affecting at least 50% of POTS patients, is a condition that impacts the small nerve fibres responsible for controlling automatic functions and sensation throughout the body. These nerve fibres manage crucial functions including temperature sensation, pain perception, sweating, and blood vessel control.

People with small fibre neuropathy often experience burning or tingling sensations, particularly in their hands and feet. They may have reduced sensitivity to temperature changes, alterations in sweating patterns, blood flow issues, and various types of pain that can be sharp, burning, or aching in nature.

The relationship between small fibre neuropathy and Dysautonomia is complex and bidirectional — each condition can affect the other, and improvements in one condition often lead to improvements in the other. This connection helps explain why many people with Dysautonomia experience temperature sensitivity, unexplained pain, or abnormal sweating patterns as part of their symptom complex.

Gastrointestinal Disorders:

Gastrointestinal (GI) issues affect approximately 30% of people with Dysautonomia, which isn't surprising given the autonomic nervous system's crucial role in controlling digestive function. These problems often manifest as nausea (particularly after eating), feeling full quickly, bloating, abdominal pain, and changes in bowel habits that can range from constipation (usually) to diarrhea or alternate between the two. Many people also experience difficulty swallowing or acid reflux.

The severity of these gastrointestinal symptoms often fluctuates and can be influenced by several factors. Symptoms frequently worsen when upright and improve when lying down — but eating or drinking safely while lying flat is easier said than done and not recommended. Meal size and osmolality play a significant role, with smaller, more frequent meals typically being better tolerated than larger ones[33]. Food temperature and overall hydration status can also impact symptom severity, as can the general state of their Dysautonomia symptoms.

Managing these gastrointestinal complications often requires a multi-faceted approach. Most people find that eating smaller, more frequent meals helps reduce symptoms. Maintaining good hydration is crucial, though this can be challenging when nausea is present (see IV saline rescue). Some people find that room temperature foods are easier to tolerate than very hot or cold items. For those with severe symptoms, working with a gastroenterologist can be beneficial. It's also worth considering whether Mast Cell Activation Syndrome might be contributing to the digestive symptoms, as these conditions frequently overlap.

---

[33] Many people with Dysautonomia feel worse after large and/or very concentrated meals because the body must move water into the digestive tract to process them. This temporary fluid shift can worsen symptoms like dizziness and fatigue. For this reason, smaller, more frequent meals are often better tolerated than large ones, and timing of larger meals should be considered carefully. Liaising with a dietician specifically about this can be useful.

Communicating About Dysautonomia and Supporting Patients

Note: As a physician, my expertise lies primarily in diagnosing conditions and managing medical treatments, including medications. Just as I strongly recommend engaging with an exercise physiologist for assistance and guidance with exercise rehabilitation, I also strongly advocate for working with a professional, trained psychologist to address the psychological impact of these debilitating, chronic, and often invisible conditions.

To provide a more comprehensive guide, I reached out to colleagues for their insights on managing the emotional and social aspects of Dysautonomia. The following section incorporates their expert advice. Any strengths in this section are a credit to their expertise, while any shortcomings are likely due to my interpretation or synthesis of the information.

This section is not a substitute for personalised psychological care. The strategies provided are general and may not be suitable for everyone. Each individual's experience with Dysautonomia is unique, and professional psychological support should be tailored to your specific needs and circumstances.

Explaining Dysautonomia to Others

Living with Dysautonomia can be challenging, and one of the most difficult aspects is often explaining your condition to friends, family, and colleagues who may not understand. Here are some strategies and tips to help you communicate effectively about your condition:

Start with the Basics

Begin by explaining that Dysautonomia is a malfunction of the autonomic nervous system (ANS). You might say:

- "My body has trouble regulating many of the automatic functions that most people don't have to think about, like heart rate, blood pressure, digestion, and temperature control."

Use Analogies

Analogies can be powerful tools for helping others understand complex concepts. Here are a few others have found useful:

- **The Faulty Thermostat**: "Imagine your body is like a house, and the ANS is the thermostat. In a normal house, the thermostat automatically adjusts to keep the temperature comfortable. In my case, the thermostat is faulty."

- **The Unreliable Assistant**: "Think of the ANS as an assistant that's supposed to handle all the background tasks in your body. For me, it's like having an unreliable assistant who sometimes doesn't show up for work — or just creates chaos."

- **The Glitchy Computer**: "My autonomic nervous system is like a computer with a glitchy operating system. Suddenly, simple tasks become difficult and unpredictable. Unfortunately, I can't turn it off and on again."

Explain Your Specific Symptoms

After providing a general explanation, describe how Dysautonomia affects you personally. For example:

- "For me, this means that when I stand up, my heart rate increases dramatically and my blood pressure drops, which can make me feel dizzy (or faint, or about to pass out)."

Address Invisible Illness

Explain that Dysautonomia is often an invisible illness:

- "Even though I might look fine on the outside, my body is working overtime to manage basic functions. This is why I might seem okay one day and be struggling the next."

Common Scenarios and How to Handle Them

Here are some specific scenarios you might encounter and suggestions for how to handle them, hopefully these get you started but it's best to work out and practice your own so they're ready to go without having to come up with something on the spot:

- **At a Social Gathering**: "I have a condition called Dysautonomia that affects my body's 'automatic' functions. Right now, my body is having trouble regulating my blood pressure when I stand for long periods. I may need to sit down or leave early to manage my symptoms."

- **At Work**: "I have a medical condition called Dysautonomia that can be unpredictable. Having the flexibility to work from home on bad days would help me manage my condition while maintaining my productivity."

- **Cancelling Plans with Friends**: "I'm really sorry, but I need to cancel our plans for tonight. My Dysautonomia is flaring up. Can we reschedule for next week?" (but I've just gotten this really great guide I hope will help!)

- **Explaining Dietary Needs**: "You might notice I'm adding extra salt and drinking a lot of water. This is actually part of managing my Dysautonomia. It helps my body maintain proper blood volume and pressure."

- **At School**:

  - For explaining to peers:
    - "My autonomic nervous system doesn't work quite right — it's like my body's software needs a major update."
    - "Some days my body handles being upright better than others."

83

- "I might need to take breaks, but it doesn't mean I'm not interested or don't want to participate."
  - For teachers/administrators:
    - "I may need to step out briefly when symptoms flare, but I'll do my best to minimise disruption."
    - "I want to participate fully, and these accommodations will help me do that."
    - "Could we discuss some flexible options for when I'm having particularly challenging days?"
  - For group work:
    - "I'm committed to doing my part, but I might need some flexibility with timing."
    - "I can contribute best by [specific task], especially on days when my symptoms are acting up."
    - "Let's have a backup plan for days when I might not be able to attend in person."

- **Explaining Exercise Limitations**: "High-intensity workouts can actually be harmful for me right now due to my Dysautonomia. I'm following a specific exercise plan designed for my condition."

- **Dating and Relationships**: "I have a chronic condition called Dysautonomia. It affects my body's 'automatic' functions, like heart rate and blood pressure. This means I sometimes have to cancel plans unexpectedly or take breaks during activities."

- **Handling Unsolicited Advice**: "I appreciate your concern and suggestion. Dysautonomia is a complex condition, and what works can vary a lot from person to person. I'm working closely with my healthcare team to manage my symptoms."

- **Explaining the Need for Mobility Aids**: "You might notice that I sometimes use a wheelchair, but other times I don't.

Dysautonomia can cause my symptoms to fluctuate, so some days I need more support than others."

- **Explaining Brain Fog**: "I'm sorry, I'm having a bit of trouble focusing right now. One of the symptoms of my Dysautonomia is something called 'brain fog'. It can make it hard for me to concentrate or find the right words sometimes."

Remember, these are just examples. Feel free to adapt them to your personal style and specific situation.

How Friends and Family Can Help Support Someone with Dysautonomia

If someone you care about has Dysautonomia, your support can make a significant difference in their quality of life. Here are some specific ways you can help:

- **Educate Yourself**: "I've been reading about Dysautonomia. I had no idea that simply standing up could be so challenging. Is that something you experience?"

- **Believe and Validate Their Experience**: "I know you said you're not feeling well today. Even though you look okay, I understand that doesn't mean you feel okay. What can I do to help?"

- **Be Flexible with Plans**: "I understand you're not feeling up to going out tonight. No worries at all. Would you like me to come over and keep you company instead, or would you prefer to rest?"

- **Offer Practical Help**: "I'm heading to the grocery store. Can I pick anything up for you while I'm there?"

- **Create a Supportive Environment**: "I've set up some chairs and water bottles in the backyard for our get-together. Let me know if you need anything else to be comfortable."

- **Listen Without Judgment**: "It sounds like you're having a really tough day. I'm here to listen if you want to talk about it."

- **Accompany Them to Medical Appointments**: "Would you like me to come with you to your next doctor's appointment? I can take notes or just be there for support." (having a second supportive person there is really helpful).

- **Encourage Self-Care**: "I know you want to push through, but it's okay to take a break. Your health comes first."

- **Include Them**: "We'd love for you to join us for dinner. We can choose a restaurant close by and with comfortable seating. If you're not feeling up to it on the day, we completely understand."

- **Learn Their Emergency Protocol**: "Can you walk me through what I should do if you faint? I want to make sure I can help if needed."

Coping with the Stress of Supporting Someone with Dysautonomia

Supporting someone with a chronic illness can be stressful. It's important to take care of your own mental health too. Here are some strategies:

- **Acknowledge Your Feelings**: "I'm feeling overwhelmed today. I know it's not anyone's fault, but I need to take some time for myself."

- **Set Boundaries**: "I care about you, but I can't be available 24/7. Let's work together to find other sources of support too."

- **Maintain Your Own Life**: "I'm going to my book club tonight. It helps me recharge so I can be more present when we're together" (and if you don't have an outside activity — find one).

- **Join a Support Group**: "I found a local support group for people whose partners have chronic illnesses. It's been really helpful to talk to others who understand."

- **Practice Self-Care**: "I'm going for a run this morning. Exercise helps me manage stress and be a better supporter."

- **Seek Professional Help**: "I've decided to start seeing a therapist. Supporting you is important to me, and I want to make sure I'm in a good place mentally to do that."

- **Educate Others**: "I've been sharing some articles about Dysautonomia with our friends. It's helping them understand what we're going through." (and maybe share sections of this really great guide you recently read…).

- **Take Breaks**: "I'm going to visit my sister this weekend. A little time away helps me recharge."

- **Celebrate Small Victories**: "You were able to go for a walk today! That's awesome. Let's celebrate with your favourite movie tonight" (with salty snacks).

- **Stay Hopeful**: "I know things are tough right now, but I'm hopeful that with continued treatment and research, things will improve."

Remember, taking care of yourself isn't selfish — it's necessary. By maintaining your own well-being, you'll be better equipped to support your loved one with Dysautonomia.

Special situations

Living with Dysautonomia means navigating many different situations, from education and work to travel and medical procedures. While not every section here will be relevant to you right now, I've tried to provide guidance for many common scenarios you might encounter.

Think of this section as a reference library — you don't need to read it all at once. Instead:

- Scan the headings to find what's relevant to your current situation.
- Bookmark sections you might need later.
- Return to other sections when they become relevant.

The situations covered include:

- Managing education.
- Returning to work.
- Pregnancy and Breastfeeding.
- IV Saline therapy.
- Surgery and medical procedures.
- Travel considerations.

Each section provides practical strategies and specific recommendations based on real experiences. Additionally, you'll find sample letters and documentation templates in the appendix that can help with many of these situations, including templates for schools, employers, travel, sports, housing, insurance and medical emergencies.

Feel free to skip past any of these that don't currently apply to you (to Some General Healthcare Advice) and focus on sections that matter most to you now, but remember — they're here if you ever need them.

Managing Education with Dysautonomia

Dysautonomia frequently disrupts studies during crucial educational years, with the potential for lifelong impacts. While managing symptoms and optimising treatment is essential, adapting the learning environment also can make a significant difference in minimising educational and social disruption. While not my area of expertise I am often asked to write letters of support so have worked with patients and their families and given the issues some thought over the years.

With appropriate accommodations and planning, most students can successfully continue their studies. You probably won't be able to get all these measures arranged, but these are accommodations others have found useful.

Documentation

Start by getting a detailed letter from your healthcare provider that includes:

- Your diagnosis and how the symptoms impact learning.
- Specific accommodations you think may help (such as below). This isn't meant to be exhaustive and if you think of something else likely to help due to local factors then it rarely hurts to ask.
- Provider's contact information for follow-up questions.

Connect with School Support

- Universities/colleges: Contact the Disability Resource Centre or Student Support Services.
- Primary/secondary schools: Speak with your guidance counsellor or school administrator.
- Schedule a meeting to discuss your needs and bring your medical documentation.

In and between Classrooms

- Permission to sit rather than stand during lengthy activities.

- Permission to keep medications that may need to be taken at specific times (e.g. pyridostigmine or midodrine) with you.
    - Set an alarm on a phone or watch to remind you to take them when due.
- Freedom to take breaks to move around or lie down when needed.
- Authorisation to keep water and salty snacks at your desk.
- Permission to wear compression garments at all times (especially with exercise).
- Temperature-controlled environments when possible.
- Elevator access if available.
- Ability to leave class briefly without drawing attention if needed without disrupting the general class.
    - Access to seats near the door for easy exits.
- Schedule classes with rest periods between them when possible.
- Choose class locations to minimise walking distances.
- Identify quiet places for rest during any free periods.
- Permission to record lectures, or use a laptop or tablet, if writing is fatiguing.

Academic Support

- Permission to have access to water and salt during test/exams.
- Extended time for tests and assignments.
- Scheduling tests for a time of day when your symptoms are typically at their best (often but not always mornings).
- Flexible attendance policies for symptom flares.
- Permission for breaks during exams.
- Access to class notes if absent.
- Ability to complete missed work at home.
- Alternative assignment formats during severe symptoms.
- Option for online or hybrid learning when available.

Physical Education and Sports

- Modified activities based on your exercise physiologist's recommendations.

- o Such as avoiding postural changes or prolonged standing still.
- Alternative options during symptom flares.
  - o Flexibility to adapt participation based on day-to-day symptom variation such as permission to sit out without penalty when necessary or the option to participate in lighter activities.
- Ready access to cold water and rest areas.
- Permission to change compression garments in private if needed.
  - o Or to have assistance to change them (they can be tight).

Managing Critical Times

- Consider IV saline loading before important study and examination periods.
- Use holiday breaks to trial new medications, minimising term-time disruption.
- Plan ahead for field trips, sports days, formals, graduations and other special events that may present special challenges but are so important to participate in if at all possible.

Communication Tips

- Keep teachers informed about your condition.
- Establish clear communication channels for difficult days.
- Be open with friends and group project members about why you may need to skip activities or take breaks sometimes.
- Practice some phrases on how to explain the situation to people in advance. More on this later.
- Build understanding early — it's much easier to say "Sorry, I'm having a really POTSie day" when friends and teachers already understand the situation.
- Update staff when your needs change.

Creating Your Support Team

- Inform trusted classmates who can help if needed.
- Work with teachers to develop make-up work protocols.
- Know who to contact for immediate assistance.

For Parents and Guardians

- Schedule regular meetings with teachers to monitor progress.
- Help develop emergency plans for severe symptoms.
- Stay actively involved in accommodation discussions.
- Maintain open communication with the school about changing needs.

Remember: Success in education while managing Dysautonomia is easier with teamwork. Work together with your healthcare team, school staff, and family to develop and adjust your plan as needed. You're not alone in this process, and with proper support and accommodations, you can achieve your educational goals while managing your health.

Returning to Work

Once you have a stable treatment plan in place, returning to work requires careful planning to avoid setbacks. While a gradual return is ideal, financial or workplace constraints may not always allow this.

Ideal Approach (if possible)

- Start with 2–3 half days per week, spaced apart to allow recovery if necessary.
- Gradually increase hours/days as tolerated.
- Consider starting with work-from-home if available.
- Build up to full duties over 4–8 weeks or longer, depending on individual response.
- Be prepared to adjust this timeline based on how your body responds.

Practical Considerations

- Minimise activities requiring prolonged standing or frequent postural changes.
- Take regular breaks to change position, hydrate/salt load, or take medications.
  - Set quiet reminders on your phone/watch if needed
  - Keep supplies at your desk/workplace.
- Consider compression garments during work hours.
  - Keep a spare pair at work if possible.
- Have a plan for managing symptom flares.
  - Identify quiet place you can lie down if needed in advance.
  - Keep if required medications readily available even if no longer regularly using them.
- Discuss necessary workplace accommodations with your employer/supervisor/HR, such as:
  - A desk or workspace close to bathrooms and break areas to minimise walking distances.
  - Ability to sit when needed.
  - Access to air conditioning.

- o Working away from heat sources.
  - o Flexibility to work from home on bad days if possible.
- Talk with co-workers in advance about your needs:
  - o That you may need to lie down sometimes.
  - o Preferred seating near air-conditioning
  - o Why you may need to leave meeting briefly
  - o How they can help in an emergency (lie you down and carefully elevate your legs).
- Manage team project expectations pro-actively:
  - o Be clear about your capabilities and limitations.
  - o Suggest tasks that play to your strengths (shouldn't everyone?)
  - o Have backup plans for bad days.
- Ensure your medications are optimised for your work schedule.
- Consider whether your role needs permanent modifications or if a change in career path might be necessary if your current position involves activities that consistently trigger symptoms.

If a gradual return isn't possible, focus on:

- Pacing yourself during work hours.
- Prioritising rest on non-work days.
- Being extra careful with symptom management (hydration, salt, compression, medications).
- Discussing with your healthcare team how to optimise your treatment plan around work demands.

Impact of Associated conditions: If you have associated conditions like MCAS, hypermobility, or ADHD, these may require additional considerations in your return-to-work plan. For example:

- People with hypermobility may need ergonomic assessments and equipment[34].
- Those with MCAS may need to focus on optimising their medication regimen and personal strategies, as workplace-

---

[34] Occupational therapists are the experts in advising on this.

wide policies (like fragrance-free environments) are rarely feasible — though it rarely hurts to ask.

- ADHD might influence how you structure your work periods and breaks.

Remember: Everyone's situation is different, and what works for one person may not work for another. Work with your healthcare providers and employer to develop a plan that fits your specific circumstances and workplace requirements. While some accommodations may not be possible, focus on what you can control and optimise — your treatment plan, personal strategies, and work patterns. Regrettably, some people may find they need to consider different roles or career paths if their original position involves activities that consistently trigger symptoms despite all treatments and accommodations.

Pregnancy

I am not an obstetrician, nor even an obstetric physician, but as Dysautonomia disproportionately affects young women I've helped manage a significant number of pregnancies in people with the condition. Pregnancy can be challenging, but with proper care and monitoring, Dysautonomia should not be a barrier to having successful pregnancies.

Changes in Symptoms

- Some women experience an improvement in Dysautonomia symptoms during pregnancy, particularly in the second trimester.
- Most however find their symptoms worsen, especially in the first and third trimesters.
- Postpartum period can be particularly challenging as the body readjusts.

Management Strategies

- **Hydration**
  - Even more crucial during pregnancy. Aim for at least 2–3 litres of fluid daily. If nausea makes this a problem, intravenous saline can be very useful.
- **Salt Intake**
  - Continue salt loading unless advised otherwise by your obstetrician.
- **Compression Garments**
  - Will need to be adjusted as your body changes, but can really help.
- **Position Changes**
  - Be extra careful when changing positions, especially later in pregnancy.
- **Exercise**
  - Continue as tolerated, focusing on exercises done while lying down or in water.

Medication Considerations

- Many medications used for Dysautonomia are considered safe during pregnancy, but always consult your healthcare provider.
- Fludrocortisone and digoxin are generally considered safe but dosing may need to be adjusted.
- Beta-blockers: Some (like metoprolol) are considered safe, while others should be avoided. I usually switch people over to labetalol as this is commonly used to manage hypertension in pregnancy and so everyone involved is familiar.
- Pyridostigmine, midodrine and ivabradine are **typically discontinued** during pregnancy due to limited safety data.

Monitoring

- More frequent prenatal visits may be necessary.
- Blood pressure and heart rate should be closely monitored.
- Some women may require fetal growth scans more frequently as determined by the obstetrician involved.

Delivery Considerations

- Discuss your delivery plan with your obstetrician and anaesthetist in advance. IV saline loading may make things smoother.
- Epidural anaesthesia is often well-tolerated and can help manage symptoms during labour.
- Have a plan for managing symptoms immediately postpartum (IV saline).

Remember, every pregnancy is unique. Work closely with your healthcare team to develop a personalised management plan that addresses both your Dysautonomia and pregnancy needs.

Breastfeeding

Key Points

Managing breastfeeding with Dysautonomia:

- Increased fluid/salt needs,
- Positioning considerations,
- Medication safety, and
- Fatigue management.

Key considerations:

- Rest during feeds,
- Consider pumping options,
- Ask for help when needed, and
- Regular monitoring.

Breastfeeding can present challenges beyond the norm for mothers with Dysautonomia. Here are some important considerations:

Hydration and Nutrition

- Breastfeeding increases fluid needs. Aim for at least 3 litres of fluid daily.
- Continue salt loading as advised by your doctor.
- Ensure adequate calorie intake to support milk production and manage symptoms.

Positioning

- Use reclined or side-lying positions to minimise orthostatic stress.
- Consider using pillows for support to reduce physical exertion.

Medication Considerations

- Many Dysautonomia medications are compatible with breastfeeding, but always consult your healthcare provider.
- Fludrocortisone, pyridostigmine, digoxin and most beta-blockers are generally considered safe.
- Midodrine and ivabradine have limited data in breastfeeding.

Managing Fatigue

- Rest during feeding sessions.
- Consider pumping to allow others to assist with feeding, especially for night feeds.

Symptom Management

- Wear compression garments during and after feeding sessions.
- Keep water and salty snacks nearby during feeds.

Support

- Don't hesitate to ask for help with positioning, bringing the baby to you, or other tasks.
- Communicate with your healthcare team about any worsening symptoms.

Remember, while breastfeeding is beneficial, it's okay to supplement with formula or switch to formula feeding if managing Dysautonomia symptoms becomes too challenging. You can't care for another if you're struggling.

Intravenous Saline Therapy

Key Points

> **As rescue therapy:**
>
> - Effective for severe flares,
> - Useful for important events, and
> - Access often challenging.
>
> **For regular use:**
>
> - Reserved for severe cases,
> - Significant commitments, and
> - Not insignificant risks and costs.

Many people with Dysautonomia report feeling significantly better for a short period after receiving intravenous (IV) saline (it's almost diagnostic), often during hospital visits for other reasons. A litre of normal saline contains 9g of salt, and hospital patients commonly receive 2–3 litres per day without issue. This dramatic improvement has led to interest in both occasional "rescue" therapy and regular infusions as a treatment option.

As Rescue Therapy: IV saline can be effective for managing severe flares or preparing for important events (like weddings or examinations). However, accessing it can be challenging outside of hospital settings. While the treatment itself is extremely safe when properly administered, regular IV access requires skilled healthcare providers and carries risks of infection or vein damage. The practical difficulties of arranging this (finding willing providers, costs, scheduling) often make it impractical for most situations. That said, if you happen to have an IV in for some other reason it's not unreasonable to request a few litres if possible.

Regular Use: Some patients with severe Dysautonomia who haven't responded well to other treatments may benefit from regular IV saline infusions (typically 2–3 litres, ranging from every few days to every couple of weeks). Whilst this can be effective, it requires:

- Careful patient selection,
- Reliable venous access (often requiring a semi-permanent line, e.g. a PICC),
- Regular monitoring,
- Experienced healthcare providers,
- Significant time commitment, and
- Substantial ongoing costs.

Choice of IV Solution: While "normal saline" (0.9% sodium chloride) is most commonly used, some clinicians prefer balanced solutions like Hartmann's/Lactated Ringer's solution or Plasmalyte, particularly for regular infusions. These better match the body's electrolyte composition and may cause less metabolic disturbance with frequent use. However, they contain less sodium than normal saline, so larger volumes may be needed for the same effect. Some centres add dextrose (sugar) to help with solution retention, though this appears to mostly help patients who also have hypoglycaemia.

The optimal choice and rate of infusion often needs to be individualised — most patients feel better with rapid infusion over a few hours, while others prefer slower administration over 4–6 hours to minimise side effects like headache or chest discomfort (these can usually be minimised by pre-warming the fluid closer to body temperature). As with many aspects of Dysautonomia management, finding the right approach often requires careful trial and monitoring.

The logistical challenges, infection risks with long-term venous access, and healthcare system constraints mean this approach is usually reserved for severe cases where all other treatments have failed. It's typically managed through specialist centres with experience in both Dysautonomia and IV infusion programs.

For most patients, focusing on oral hydration, salt loading, and other standard treatments remains more practical and safer for long-term management. However, knowing that IV saline can be beneficial helps explain why aggressive oral fluid and salt intake is so important in day-to-day management.

Surgery

Key Points

Pre-surgery preparation:

- Inform all healthcare providers,
- Review medications,
- Plan fluid management, and
- Discuss anaesthesia needs.

Recovery focus:

- Careful mobilisation,
- Return to compression,
- Symptom monitoring,
- Medication adjustment, and
- Symptom management strategies.

If you have Dysautonomia and are facing surgery, there are a few considerations to keep in mind:

Pre-operative Considerations

- **Medication Management**
  - Discuss all your medications with your anaesthetist and surgeon.
  - Some medications may need to be adjusted or temporarily stopped before surgery.
- **Hydration**
  - Maintaining proper hydration is crucial, especially whilst fasting before the procedure.
  - I recommend a 2–3L IV saline (or similar) load before and over the operation if possible as things tend to go smoother.

- **Anxiety Management**
  - Discuss strategies to manage pre-operative anxiety, which can exacerbate symptoms.

During Surgery

- **Anaesthesia**
  - Inform your anaesthetist about your Dysautonomia.
  - They may need to adjust their protocols to prevent blood pressure fluctuations.
- **Position**
  - The surgical team should be aware of potential issues with prolonged supine positioning.
- **Temperature Regulation**
  - Extra attention may be needed to maintain body temperature.

Post-operative Considerations

- **Pain Management**
  - Some pain medications can affect blood pressure and heart rate.
  - Work with your care team to find the right balance.
- **Mobilisation**
  - Early but careful mobilisation is important to prevent blood pooling.
  - Take your time first slowly sitting up and making sure you're okay before standing or walking the first couple of times after the procedure.
  - Consider using compression garments as soon as possible post-surgery (not just the usual stockings to the knees used by hospitals to stop clots developing, but your own proper grade 2, ankle/knee to waist compression garment). Obviously, this doesn't apply if it will be an issue with any wounds or drains, depending on the nature of the surgery.
- **Hydration and Electrolytes**
  - Continued attention to hydration and electrolyte balance is crucial.

- **Symptom Monitoring**
  - Be vigilant for any worsening of Dysautonomia symptoms post-surgery.

Remember to communicate clearly with your entire healthcare team about your Dysautonomia. Consider having a letter from your Dysautonomia specialist to share with the surgical team (even just "Xxxxxx has Dysautonomia, everyone's lives will likely go easier if you pre-load them with 2–3L of IV saline perioperatively"). With proper planning and awareness, usually even major surgeries and their recovery are no more of an issue than for people without the issue.

Travel

Key Points

Travel management:

- Wear compression during travel,
- Maintain hydration,
- Plan regular movement, and
- Choose appropriate seating.

Practical considerations:

- Accommodation selection,
- Medication timing,
- Rest periods, and
- Symptom management strategies.

Prolonged travel (especially flights, but also car and train trips) can be challenging for people with Dysautonomia due to prolonged sitting, dehydration, and changes in air pressure. Here are some strategies to make your journey more comfortable:

Before the trip

- **Compression Gear**
  - Wear compression stockings, garments or a binder. This is the major tip.
- **Choose Your Seat**
  - Book an aisle seat for easy access to the bathroom and to stretch your legs.
- **Book accommodation at a place with an elevator or on the ground floor**
  - Preferably with air conditioning too.

During the trip

- **Stay Hydrated**
  - Drink plenty of water and (strongly) consider cold electrolyte drinks.
- **Move Regularly**
  - Walk a bit every hour if possible, or do seated exercises.
- **Elevate Your Feet**
  - Use a footrest or your carry-on bag to elevate your feet as much as practical. Book a seat with extra legroom to help with this if possible.
- **Avoid Alcohol and Caffeine**
  - These can worsen dehydration and symptoms.
- **Eat Small, Frequent Meals**
  - This can help stabilise blood sugar and reduce nausea.
- **Inform attendants about your condition**
  - If you're concerned about managing symptoms during a bus trip, flight or at a hotel.
- **Ask for help if needed**
  - Better to ask early for help then to regret not asking once it's too late.

Managing Symptoms

- **Dizziness**
  - Recline your seat, or lie down if possible, if feeling lightheaded.
- **Nausea**
  - Use acupressure bands or ask for ginger ale.
- **Fatigue**
  - Bring earplugs and an eye mask to help you rest.

After the trip

- **Take It Slow**
  - Allow time to adjust before standing and again before walking.

- **Rehydrate**
  - Continue to drink fluids (and salt) after the trip.
- **Rest**
  - If possible, plan for rest time after your trip before any activities.

With proper planning, people with even severe Dysautonomia can travel successfully, even by air.

Some General Healthcare Advice

Privacy and Medical Records

Managing Your Medical Information

- Keep detailed records of your symptoms, test results, and treatments. This helps ensure continuity of care and can be valuable when seeing new healthcare providers.
- Consider keeping a medical diary documenting:
    - Symptoms and their severity,
    - Medication responses and side effects,
    - Test results and medical reports, and
    - Names and contact details of your healthcare providers.

Privacy Considerations

- Your medical information is protected by privacy laws. In Australia, this includes the Privacy Act 1988 and various state/territory health records laws.
- You have the right to:
    - Access your medical records,
    - Request corrections to your records,
    - Control who has access to your health information, and
    - Complain if your privacy is breached.
- When sharing your medical information:
    - Be cautious about sharing details on social media or public forums,
    - Only share what's necessary with employers or schools,
    - Keep copies of important medical documents in a secure location, and
    - Consider who has access to any health apps or digital records you use.

International Considerations

Reminder: The management approaches described in this guide are based primarily on Australian medical practice and may differ in other countries. Important considerations include:

Medication Availability

- Medications mentioned may:
    - Not be available in all countries.
    - Have different brand names internationally.
    - Have different costs or subsidy arrangements.
    - Need different dosage forms or strengths.

Healthcare Systems

- Access to specialists and treatments varies significantly between countries.
- Funding models and costs differ internationally.
- Some treatments may require different approvals or qualifications.
- Waiting times and referral processes vary by location.

Conclusion

Key Principles to Remember

Recovery is Possible

- Proper treatment can speed recovery.
- Everyone's journey is different.
- Good days and bad days are normal, the aim is for more and better good days over time.

Treatment Fundamentals

- Appropriate exercise is (currently) the only proven way to improve recovery time.
- Other treatments help you feel better day-to-day.
- "Start low and go slow" with medications.
- Most people need a combination of approaches.
- What works is proven for a reason
- Finding what works for you is more important than what "should" work.

Managing Your Care

- Build a partnership with your healthcare team.
- You can't benefit from treatments you don't try.
- Save time and money by focusing on what's known to work.
- Keep track of what helps you feel better.

- Be wisely sceptical of expensive "miracle cures".
- Be patient finding your right treatment mix.
- Adjust treatments as your needs change.
- If something isn't helping, there are many other options to try.

Living with Dysautonomia

- A little planning can make a big difference.
- Listen to your body.
- Track your progress — memory can be unreliable with brain fog.
- Use your tools (compression, hydration, medications).
- Connect with supportive people.
- Celebrate improvements, even the small ones.

Remember: While Dysautonomia can be challenging, understanding and managing it well can help you get back to enjoying life. You're not alone on this journey, and there are many different ways to work toward feeling better.

Dysautonomias can greatly affect people during what are usually seen as some of the most important years of their lives. However, with the right understanding and treatments, there is hope for real improvements in their quality of life. I hope this guide and the resources that come with it will help make that process quicker and easier.

After this Conclusion are organisational directories, diagnostic tools, detailed medication guides and treatment protocols, various letter templates and a comprehensive glossary — all designed to support you and your healthcare team in your treatment journey.

If you found this guide helpful in understanding and managing Dysautonomia, please consider sharing it with others who might benefit — whether they're fellow patients, healthcare providers, or support groups. Personal recommendations and positive reviews are invaluable in helping this information reach those who need it most, particularly on platforms where others are searching for reliable resources about Dysautonomia.

The current intention is for new editions to be released periodically as practice-changing developments in the field occur, ensuring the information remains current and useful. The latest edition information and printable versions of most subsequent resources are available at **https://aionhealth.com.au/dysautonomia-resources.**

Dysautonomia-Specific Organisations and Websites

Dysautonomia International:
www.dysautonomiainternational.org

A US based not-for-profit patient advocacy group focusing on research, education, and patient support for those affected by various forms of Dysautonomia, including POTS. They provide resources for patients, caregivers, and healthcare professionals. Regularly updates their website with new research. Has specific chapters in a number of other countries, along with a very large Facebook group and numerous different support groups.

Standing up to POTS: standinguptopots.org

US based more medically lead non-profit organisation dedicated to improving the quality of life for people with POTS specifically through research, advocacy, and support

PoTS UK: potsuk.org

UK based charity that focuses on supporting individuals affected by POTS.

Australian POTS Foundation: potsfoundation.org.au

A non-profit dedicated to improving outcomes for those with POTS through advocacy, support, and research. They aim to raise funds for research, education, and support for the POTS community in Australia[35].

New Zealand Dysautonomia Support:

A Facebook support group for individuals with Dysautonomia conditions like POTS in New Zealand. They provide peer support and share information.

---

[35] I'm not on their practitioner list as I'm already overworked and not looking for more.

Wikipedia — Postural Orthostatic Tachycardia Syndrome:
wikipedia.org/wiki/Postural_orthostatic_tachycardia_syndrome

A pretty good guide that has gone through a few evolutions over the last decade.

My biggest criticism of the current version[36] is that it implies that you will have a certain subtype and that certain therapies will thus be reliably effective. Again, I wish it was that simple.

---

[36] January 2025.

Associated Conditions Organisations and Websites

Select organisations that provide comprehensive international resources for conditions commonly associated with Dysautonomia:

Ehlers-Danlos Syndrome (EDS)

- **The Ehlers-Danlos Society**: www.ehlers-danlos.com
  - The premier global resource for EDS, offers comprehensive educational materials, research updates, and support networks accessible worldwide.

Mast Cell Disorders

- **The Mastocytosis Society**: www.tmsforacure.org
  - While US-based, their extensive educational resources and research information make them a valuable international reference for mast cell disorders, including MCAS.

ADHD and Autism

- **CHADD**: www.chadd.org
  - Provides resources for comprehensive training programs and science-based information about ADHD.
- **Autistic Self Advocacy Network**: www.autisticadvocacy.org
  - Autistic-led organisation advancing disability rights and providing resources for understanding autism.

Endometriosis

- **Endometriosis Association**: www.endometriosisassn.org
  - International organisation pioneering research and providing comprehensive educational resources.

Migraines

- **International Headache Society**: www.ihs-headache.org
  - Global organisation advancing headache science and providing evidence-based resources.

This guide is focussed on Dysautonomia, so while these associated conditions are important to acknowledge, providing a comprehensive list of support organisations for each condition in every country would quickly become a book in itself. To find local support organisations in your area, consider discussing this with your healthcare provider or searching online using terms specific to your location.

Resources and handouts

The following various resources, guides and sample letter templates are also available in A4 .pdf format to make them easier to print and share at:

https://aionhealth.com.au/dysautonomia-resources

Common Symptoms of Dysautonomia and POTS

- ☐ Fatigue
- ☐ Exercise intolerance
- ☐ Light-headedness/dizziness upon standing (pre-syncope)
- ☐ Fainting upon standing (syncope)
- ☐ "Brain fog" and difficulty concentrating
- ☐ Sleep disturbances
- ☐ Headaches
- ☐ Rapid heart rate (tachycardia) when standing up
- ☐ Awareness of heart beating (palpitations)
- ☐ Gastrointestinal issues like nausea, bloating, diarrhea, or constipation
- ☐ Subjective shortness of breath
- ☐ Difficulty tolerating an upright posture (orthostatic intolerance)
- ☐ Tremors
- ☐ Excessive thirst — usually to the degree that people carry water with them
- ☐ Sweating abnormalities (excessive or insufficient sweating)
- ☐ Mood swings, anxiety, and depression
- ☐ Skin sensitivity, pins and needles, or temperature dysregulation — usually above the waist
- ☐ Bladder issues like frequent urination
- ☐ Chest pain
- ☐ Weakness
- ☐ Blurred vision
- ☐ Chest discomfort

The hallmark features are light-headedness, dizziness, and fainting upon standing up, along with a rapid heart rate. Other common symptoms include fatigue, brain fog, nausea, headaches, and gastrointestinal issues.

This is a long list, and most things on it have many potential causes. Just because you have one (or even a lot) of these symptoms does not mean you have a Dysautonomia.

Fortunately, very few people will have all or even most of the symptoms listed, but if you have a number of them, it is worth considering that maybe Dysautonomia may be causative and investigating further.

Pulse Rate and Blood Pressure Orthostatic Variation Tracking

Instructions: Record your blood pressure (BP) and pulse rate per minute twice daily — once in the morning and once in the evening. Take readings first after lying down for a few minutes and then after standing up. Use the comments section to note how you're feeling or any factors that might affect your readings.

Note: The exact timing of when you take the standing measurement isn't critical — precise timing only matters in borderline cases, and even then, if your symptoms and story suggest Dysautonomia, treatment may still be worth trying even if you don't meet the strict diagnostic criteria.

The cost of a BP machine can vary significantly between countries. It's often worthwhile to see if an older relative has one you can borrow for a couple of weeks or a local pharmacy may rent them out.

Date	Time	Position	BP (mmHg)	Pulse (bpm)	Comments
/ /20__	Morning	Lying	/	___	
		Standing	/	___	
	Evening	Lying	/	___	
		Standing	/	___	
/ /20__	Morning	Lying	/	___	
		Standing	/	___	
	Evening	Lying	/	___	
		Standing	/	___	
/ /20__	Morning	Lying	/	___	
		Standing	/	___	

	Evening	Lying	/	___	
		Standing	/	___	
/ /20__	Morning	Lying	/	___	
		Standing	/	___	
	Evening	Lying	/	___	
		Standing	/	___	
/ /20__	Morning	Lying	/	___	
		Standing	/	___	
	Evening	Lying	/	___	
		Standing	/	___	
/ /20__	Morning	Lying	/	___	
		Standing	/	___	
	Evening	Lying	/	___	
		Standing	/	___	
/ /20__	Morning	Lying	/	___	
		Standing	/	___	
	Evening	Lying	/	___	
		Standing	/	___	
/ /20__	Morning	Lying	/	___	
		Standing	/	___	
	Evening	Lying	/	___	
		Standing	/	___	

Note: BP is recorded as systolic/diastolic (e.g. 120/80mmHg).

If you notice any consistently high BP readings (over 140/80mmHg, please consult your healthcare provider.

125

Fludrocortisone (Florinef) Usage Guide for Dysautonomia

General Information

- Tablet strength: 100mcg (0.1mg), scored for easy halving.
- Store in refrigerator (2–8°C or 36–46°F).
- Mechanism: Increases sodium retention in kidneys, leading to water retention and potassium excretion by mimicking the hormone aldosterone.
- A pure mineralocorticoid analogue, so whilst many people are cautious about glucocorticoid steroid effects as it ends in "cortisone" these are not a factor unless at very, very, high doses.

Dosage Protocol

Start low and increase gradually every 5–7 days until improvement or side effects occur:

- 50mcg (1/2 tablet) daily for one week, then

- 100mcg (1 tablet) daily for one week, then

- 150mcg (1 1/2 tablets) daily for one week, then

- 200mcg (2 tablets) daily for one week, then

- 250mcg (2 1/2 tablets) daily for one week, then

- 300mcg (3 tablets) daily.

Stop increasing when you feel sufficient improvement, or after reaching 300mcg with no effect.

Note: Higher doses can be used but will need medical supervision for monitoring of blood potassium levels.

Side Effects

Common: Fluid retention, bloating, headache, stomach ache.

If side effects occur:

- Skip 1–2 doses until recovered.
- Return to the last effective dose without side effects.

Important Notes

- Potassium levels: Generally, not a concern below 300mcg daily, unless on an unusual diet.
- If no improvement at 300mcg, discontinue and explore other options.
- Doses above 300mcg: Consult a doctor and monitor serum potassium levels closely.
- Take with food or milk to reduce stomach upset.

Monitoring

- Regular blood pressure checks.
- Periodic blood tests to check electrolyte levels, especially potassium.
- Weight monitoring (sudden weight gain may indicate fluid retention).

Dietary Considerations

- Maintain a consistent salt intake in your diet.
- Increase potassium-rich foods if recommended by your doctor.

For Medical Practitioners

- Consider potassium supplementation for doses exceeding 300mcg.
- Some patients may benefit from higher doses with careful monitoring.
- Regularly assess effectiveness and side effects.
- Be aware of potential drug interactions, especially with other medications affecting electrolyte balance.

Precautions

- Inform all healthcare providers about this medication.

- Discuss use during pregnancy or breastfeeding with a doctor, though most obstetricians are happy for it to be continued.

Remember: Adjust treatment based on individual patient response and always prioritise patient safety. If unusual or severe side effects occur, cease the medication and report them to your healthcare provider immediately.

Beta-Blockers Usage Guide for Dysautonomia

General Information

- Common agents: Propranolol (Inderal or Deralin), Bisoprolol (Bicor), Atenolol (Noten), or other beta-blockers.
- Well-known class of medications familiar to all doctors.
- Mechanism: Works by slowing the pulse.
- Paradoxical effect in POTS: May improve symptoms despite lowering blood pressure.

Important Notes

- Not generally suitable for people with asthma (though some types that mainly act on the heart rather than the lungs may be safe in mild to moderate asthma cases — this will be considered by the prescribing doctor).
- If you feel notably worse in any way, stop taking and discuss with your doctor.
- The ideal is to feel better, not worse.
- If no benefit is observed, try other treatments.
- May reduce blood volume, which can be a concern for people with hypovolemic POTS (a type where the body has trouble maintaining enough blood volume).

Common Side Effects

- Apathy.
- Nightmares.
- Erectile dysfunction.
- Excessive heart rate slowing.
- Dizziness on standing (may paradoxically improve in POTS).

Propranolol Protocol

Advantages: Well-studied in POTS, affordable, may reduce migraine frequency.

Disadvantages: Can negatively impact the effect of some ADHD medications.

Dosage: 10mg tablets, and 40mg tablets available for higher doses.
Increase every 3–5 days as follows:

Days	Morning Dose	Evening Dose
1–3+	1 tablet	1 tablet
4–6+	2 tablets	2 tablets
7–9+	3 tablets	3 tablets
10–12+	4 tablets	4 tablets

Note: Increase dose only if needed and well-tolerated. Do not exceed recommended maximum dose without discussing with your doctor first.

Bisoprolol Protocol

Advantages: Affordable, doesn't get into the brain well (less apathy and nightmares), can be only once a day.

Disadvantages: Not as well studied in POTS, won't help migraine.

Dosage forms: 2.5mg, 5mg and 10mg tablets
Increase every 3–5 days as follows:

Days	Morning Dose	Evening Dose
1–3+	2.5mg	2.5mg
4–6+	5mg	5mg
7–9+	7.5mg	7.5mg
10–12+	10mg	10mg

Note: Increase dose only if needed and well-tolerated. Do not exceed recommended maximum dose without discussing with your doctor first.

Very, very, few people will get to the 20mg total a day, but for a minority that is what it takes.

Once twice a day dosing is established, if desired you can try taking it all at once daily (i.e. instead of 5mg twice a day, just take 10mg of a morning) and see it that works just as well and is simpler. If it doesn't work as well then go back to the divided dosing.

Additional Considerations

- **Combination Therapy**: Very little point in taking both a beta-blocker and ivabradine as they both work to slow the heart. However, in some cases where each agent is dose-limited by side effects, a combination of two agents at low doses may be successful.
- **Monitoring**: Regular heart rate and blood pressure checks.
- **Gradual Discontinuation**: Do not stop suddenly; taper off.
- **Drug Interactions**: Inform all healthcare providers about this medication.
- **Pregnancy/Breastfeeding**: Discuss risks and benefits with your doctor (Labetalol is generally the preferred beta-blocking agent in pregnancy and it's relatively easy to convert across).
- **Diabetes**: Can mask symptoms of low blood sugar; monitor glucose levels carefully.
- **Asthma**: Use with caution in patients with respiratory conditions.

For Medical Practitioners

- Consider combining low doses of beta-blockers with ivabradine in select cases where each agent is dose-limited by side effects.
- Be aware of potential interactions with psychiatric or ADHD medications, especially for propranolol.
- Educate patients on recognising signs of excessive beta-blockade (e.g. bradycardia, hypotension).

Remember: Individualise treatment based on patient response and always prioritise patient safety.

Ivabradine (Coralan) Usage Guide for Dysautonomia

General Information

- Available as 5mg and 7.5mg tablets.
- Mechanism: Specifically slows the heart's natural pacemaker.
- Particularly beneficial for hyperadrenergic variant of POTS and for some with Long COVID.
- Goal: Regulate heart rate to a more normal level.

Dosage Protocol

Increase dose every 3 days until finding the right dose for you.

If you step up the dose and feel worse, then stop until improved and then go back to whatever was the best dose for you.

Days	Morning Dose	Evening Dose
1–3	½ tablet (2.5mg)	½ tablet (2.5mg)
4–6	1 tablet (5mg)	1 tablet (5mg)
7–9	1½ tablets (7.5mg)	1½ tablets (7.5mg)
10 onwards	2 tablets (10mg)	2 tablets (10mg)

Notes:

- You should feel a bit better with each step up until you reach either "enough" or "too much" (i.e. you feel worse).
- If not noticing any improvement by the highest dose in the table, discontinue use.
- Discuss with a doctor before exceeding the doses listed above.
- In rare cases, doses as high as 22.5mg twice a day have been used to achieve proper control.
- Once the optimal dose is determined, to save on the cost and pill burden, many people will be able to manage with halving the night time dose as they are lying down overnight.

Side Effects

Most common: Visual changes

- Typical symptoms: Lights seem very bright, "comet tails" on lights.
- Action: Stop medication if these occur.
- Can return to the highest dose that didn't cause side effects once visual changes resolve, if benefits are sufficient.

Important Considerations

- **Pregnancy**: Not recommended during pregnancy or when trying to conceive.
- **Monitoring**: Regular heart rate checks to ensure appropriate response.
- **Gradual Discontinuation**: Consult your doctor before stopping the medication.
- **Drug Interactions**: Inform all healthcare providers about this medication.
- **Individual Response**: Effects may vary; close monitoring is essential.

For Medical Practitioners

- Consider Ivabradine particularly for patients with hyperadrenergic POTS.
- Be aware that some patients may require doses higher than standard recommendations.
- Monitor for visual side effects and adjust dosage accordingly.
- Educate patients on recognising both beneficial effects and potential side effects.
- Consider combination therapy with low-dose beta-blockers in select cases where each agent is dose-limited by side effects.

Remember: Individualise treatment based on patient response and always prioritise patient safety.

Pyridostigmine (Mestinon) Usage Guide for Dysautonomia

General Information

- Available as:
    - 10mg tablets (immediate release).
    - 60mg tablets (immediate release, can be halved).
    - 180mg tablets (slow release, can be halved).
- Mechanism: Inhibits breakdown of acetylcholine, magnifying parasympathetic effects ("Boosts the vagus nerve").
- Effect typically lasts about 4 hours (may vary).

Dosage Protocol

Start with 10mg every 4 hours as needed during awake hours (e.g. 7am, 11am, 3pm).

Increase in 10mg steps every 3 days until reaching 60mg, then continue in 30mg increments.

Work the dose up until either "good enough" or side effects. If side effects occur then drop back down to whatever dose you found most effective:

Days	Dose per 4 hours when active through the day
1–3	10mg
4–6	20mg
7–9	30mg
10–12	40mg
13–15	50mg
16–18	60mg
19–21	90mg
22–24	120mg
25–27	150mg
28–30	180mg

Notes:

- Usually the most effective dose range is between 20–60mg per dose.
  - Some patients may benefit from doses as low as 10mg or as high as 180mg.
- Can adjust dosage based on daily needs (e.g. different morning vs. afternoon doses).
- Continue increasing until you find the optimal balance of benefits and side effects.
- If a dose works well, maintain that dosage.

Timing Considerations

- Typical dosing times: Upon waking (e.g. 7am), mid-morning (11am), mid-afternoon (3pm).
- Evening dose optional based on individual needs.
- Not typically taken before bed (effects less necessary while lying down/sleeping).
- Effects usually felt about 20 minutes after taking, lasting about 4 hours.

Side Effects

Common side effects to watch for:

- Abdominal discomfort or cramps.
- Excess saliva production.
- Increased bowel frequency.

Note: Side effects typically last only about 4 hours.

Contraindications

- Hypersensitivity to pyridostigmine or bromides.
- Mechanical intestinal or urinary obstruction.
- Caution in patients with bronchial asthma, seizures, or bradycardia.

Important Considerations

- **Optimal Dosing**: Don't settle for "good enough" — try the next dose level to find the best effect.

- **Individual Response**: Effects and optimal dosage may vary significantly between individuals.
- **Gradual Increase**: Keep increasing dose if no effect is seen, up to 180mg per dose.
- **Consultation**: Discuss with your doctor if high doses (90–180mg) produce no effect or side effects. Usually if no effect at this dose then cease, but it is unusual to have no effect either way at this dose and may prompt further investigation.
- **Flexibility**: Dosage can be adjusted based on daily activities and symptoms.

Special Populations

- Use during pregnancy and breastfeeding should be discussed with a healthcare provider.

For Medical Practitioners

- Encourage patients to find their optimal dose through careful titration.
- Be aware of the wide range of effective doses (10–180mg per dose).
- Monitor for gastrointestinal side effects and adjust dosage accordingly.
- Educate patients on the importance of timing doses throughout the day.

Remember: Individualise treatment based on patient response and always prioritise patient safety.

Midodrine (Vasodrine) Usage Guide for Dysautonomia

General Information

- Available as 2.5mg, 5mg, and 10mg tablets.
- Mechanism: Alpha$_1$ sympathetic agonist that causes blood vessel constriction.
- Effect typically lasts about 3.5 hours (may vary).

Dosage Protocol

Start with 2.5mg per dose for a few days, then increase as tolerated and required.

Example dosing schedule:

Days	Dose ever few hours as required
1–3	2.5mg
4–6	5mg
7–9	7.5mg
10+	10mg

Notes:

- Increase dose gradually based on individual response and tolerance.
- Some patients may benefit from doses as high as 15mg up to 4 times a day (in severe cases, under careful medical supervision).
- Subsequent doses in a day may be effective at half the initial dose.

Timing Considerations

- First dose: Take upon waking, before getting out of bed.
  - Keep medication and water by bedside.
  - Wait 15–20 minutes after taking for it to take effect before getting up.
- Subsequent doses: Take as needed, typically every 3–3.5 hours.

- Some may only need it before exercise or prolonged upright periods.

Side Effects

Common side effects to watch for:

- Hairs standing on end.
- Tingling scalp and/or neck.
- Rarely: headache.

Note: Comes with a warning not to lie down for some hours after taking. This is primarily a concern for people with Parkinson's disease and is less relevant for typical younger Dysautonomia patients without this condition.

Contraindications

- Severe organic heart disease.
- Acute renal disease.
- Urinary retention.
- Phaeochromocytoma.
- Thyrotoxicosis.

Special Populations

- Use during pregnancy and breastfeeding should be discussed with a healthcare provider.
- Caution in elderly patients due to increased risk of supine hypertension.

Important Considerations

- **Individual Response**: Effects and optimal dosage may vary significantly between individuals.
- **Gradual Increase**: Start low and increase dose slowly as needed.
- **Flexible Dosing**: Can be used as needed or on a regular schedule depending on symptoms.
- **Onset of Action**: Effects usually felt about 15–20 minutes after taking.
- **Duration**: Effects typically last 3–3.5 hours.

For Medical Practitioners

- Encourage patients to find their optimal dose through careful titration.
- Be aware of the wide range of effective doses (1.25mg to 15mg per dose).
- Monitor for side effects and adjust dosage accordingly.
- Consider this medication particularly effective for orthostatic hypotension in Dysautonomia.
- Educate patients on the importance of timing doses throughout the day.
- For severe cases, doses up to 15mg 4 times daily may be considered with close monitoring.

Remember: Individualise treatment based on patient response and always prioritise patient safety.

Digoxin for Dysautonomia: A Clinical Guide

Background

- Digoxin (Sigmaxin or Lanoxin): Available as 62.5mcg or 250mcg tablets.
- Traditionally used for atrial fibrillation or heart failure.
- Very limited published evidence for POTS: One study showed promising results in tilt table tests.
- Clinical experience suggests variable efficacy: ineffective for some, highly effective for others.
- Consider as a later-line option after standard treatments have been tried.

Dosing and Monitoring

- Starting dose: 62.5mcg each morning for 1 week,
- Increase to 125mcg each morning for 1 week,
- Check blood level after 1 week on 125mcg per day.

IMPORTANT: Blood test must be taken in the morning BEFORE taking that day's dose. We need the trough level, not the peak.

Interpreting Results and Next Steps

	Low Blood Level	Therapeutic Blood Level
No Symptom Change	Increase dose, recheck level in 1 week	Discontinue and try alternative treatment
Symptom Improvement	Consider dose increase for potential additional benefit	Continue current dose

Important Notes

- Target blood level range: Same as for other indications (to avoid toxicity).

- Main side effects: Nausea and loss of appetite.
- Pregnancy/Breastfeeding: Can be safely used.
- Renal function: Use caution in severe kidney failure (rare in POTS patients).
- Discontinuation: Can be stopped abruptly; effects wear off in 5–7 days.

Clinical Pearls

- Efficacy varies widely among patients.
- No known predictive factors for response.
- Consider as a later-line option when standard treatments have failed.
- Thoroughly explain the off-label use and limited evidence base to patients.

Remember: This guide is based on limited evidence and clinical experience. Always use clinical judgment and consider individual patient factors when prescribing.

Mast Cell Activation Syndrome (MCAS): A Patient's Guide

What is MCAS?

MCAS is a condition where your mast cells (a type of immune cell) become overactive, leading to various symptoms that can affect multiple parts of your body.

Common Symptoms

- Skin issues (rashes, itching).
- Respiratory problems (frequent sinusitis, hay fever-like symptoms).
- Gastrointestinal issues (food sensitivities, gut pain, heartburn, nausea, vomiting, diarrhea).
- Other symptoms may include headaches, fatigue, and mild cognitive problems.

Diagnosis

Diagnosing MCAS can be challenging. Your doctor may diagnose an "MCAS-like" condition based on your symptoms and response to treatment, even without formal testing.

Treatment Trial

Your doctor may suggest a treatment trial using a combination of two types of antihistamine medications:

- One H1 Blocker (available over-the-counter):
  Choose ONE of the following, to be taken twice daily at twice the standard dose:
  - Fexofenadine: 360mg
  - Cetirizine: 20mg
  - Levocetirizine: 10mg
  - Loratadine: 20mg
  - Desloratadine: 10mg

PLUS

- One H2 Blocker (usually requires a prescription):
  Choose ONE of the following, to be taken twice daily:

142

- Famotidine: 40mg
- Nizatidine: 300mg

You'll try one medication from each category at the same time for 1–2 weeks.

What to Expect

- Initial Response: After starting the treatment, observe how your symptoms change over 1–2 weeks.

- If Very Effective:

  - For the over-the-counter H1 Blocker: You may gradually reduce the dose to find the lowest amount that still manages your symptoms effectively.
  - For the prescription H2 Blocker: Consult with your doctor before making any changes.

- If Partially Effective:

  - For the H1 Blocker: You might try switching to a different option from the list to see if one works better for you.
  - For the H2 Blocker: Discuss with your doctor about possibly trying the other option.

- If Minimally Effective: Your doctor might suggest additional medications or different approaches.

- Ongoing Management:

  - Keep track of your symptoms and how they respond to different medications and doses.
  - You may find that you need to adjust your medication (especially the H1 Blocker) based on symptom flare-ups or improvements.
  - Always inform your doctor about any changes you make to your treatment plan.

Remember, everyone's experience with MCAS is different. Be patient and communicate openly with your healthcare team about your symptoms and response to treatment. While you have some flexibility with the over-the-counter medication, always consult your doctor before making significant changes to your treatment plan, especially with prescription medications.

Mast Cell Activation Syndrome (MCAS): A Guide for Medical Practitioners

Overview

MCAS, first proposed in 2010, is an umbrella term describing inappropriate mast cell activation. As of 2022, it includes both primary and secondary mast cell disorders.

Diagnostic Criteria

All three must be met:

1. Episodic, objective signs/symptoms involving ≥2 organ systems: skin, respiratory, gastrointestinal, or cardiovascular.

2. Evidence of systemic mast cell-mediator release, temporally corresponding with symptoms.

   o Serum tryptase increase: (1.2 x baseline) + 2 ng/mL.

   o Alternative mediators: >100% increase above baseline and exceeding normal range.

3. Response to mast cell-targeted medications.

Practical Approach

- Formal criteria can be challenging to meet, especially capturing an elevated serum tryptase.
- Similarly, for many people the symptoms are either continual due to ongoing chronic allergen exposure, or not objectively apparent (e.g. upper GI involvement).
- Alternatively, consider an "MCAS-like" diagnosis based on symptoms and treatment response. Given the significant chance of the patient improving with safe, simple and cheap medications, where's the harm in a temporary treatment trial?
- Common symptoms: food sensitivities, GI issues, rashes, flushing, itching, sinusitis/hay fever symptoms, Dysautonomia.

145

- Note: Headache, fatigue, cognitive issues overlap with POTS symptoms.

Treatment Trial

Initiate a combination therapy using one medication from each category:

1. H1 Blocker (non-sedating) — Choose one:
   Administer twice daily at twice the standard dosing

Medication	Dose
Fexofenadine	360mg BD
Cetirizine	20mg BD
Levocetirizine	10mg BD
Loratadine	20mg BD
Desloratadine	10mg BD

PLUS

2. H2 Blocker — Choose one:

Medication	Dose
Famotidine	40mg BD
Nizatidine	300mg BD

Trial the selected combination for 1–2 weeks.

Treatment Considerations

- If the initial combination is very effective, gradually taper doses to find the lowest effective dose/combination that adequately manages symptoms.
- If partially effective, consider rotating through options within each medication class to identify the most effective agent for the individual patient.
- If still inadequate symptom control, consider adding:

146

- Ketotifen: Start at 0.5mg BD, titrate up to 2mg BD over weeks.
- Montelukast: 10mg daily.
- Cromolyn: standard dosing.
- If ineffective, discontinue and consider alternative diagnoses.

Follow-up

- Adjust dosages based on symptom control.
- Consider referral to an immunologist for complex cases or if the above treatments are insufficiently effective.

Remember: This approach is based on clinical experience. Always use professional judgment and consider individual patient factors when diagnosing and treating.

Templates/Sample Documentation

Personally, I dislike writing letters to a school, employers and such as I often feel I'm being asked to comment on areas outside my expertise.

The following letters provide templates that healthcare providers can use or adapt when documenting accommodation needs for people with Dysautonomia. While not every patient will need every accommodation listed, these samples attempt to be comprehensive templates that can be customised based on individual circumstances and requirements.

These are deliberately detailed, as it's easier to remove irrelevant sections than to know what to add. As different situations will require different levels of detail or emphasis they can be modified based on:

- Individual patient needs,
- Local requirements,
- Specific circumstances, or
- Particular institutional policies.

The suggested approach is to focus on explaining the medical condition and its impacts, while suggesting (rather than prescribing) accommodations that others have found helpful. The final decisions about specific accommodations should be made through discussion between the patient and the institution involved, based on their particular circumstances and capabilities. I also recommend running any proposed letter by the patient for their input before official release.

I have included sample templates for:

- School/University,
- Employment,
- Travel,
- Sport/Exercise,
- Insurance/Disability,

- Housing, and
- Emergency Information.

These letters, along with other resources from this guide, are available in editable .pdf format at http://aionhealth.com.au/dysautonomia-resources for easy copying into your preferred word processing software.

School:

[Date]

RE: Educational Considerations for [Student Name] DOB: [Date of Birth]

To Whom It May Concern:

I am writing regarding my patient, [Student Name], who has Postural Orthostatic Tachycardia Syndrome (POTS), a form of Dysautonomia. This medical condition affects the autonomic nervous system, which controls involuntary body functions including heart rate, blood pressure, and temperature regulation.

Medical Impact on Learning: [Student Name]'s condition causes symptoms that can affect their educational participation in the following ways:

- Physical symptoms including dizziness and fatigue can make prolonged standing difficult.
- Blood pressure regulation issues can cause problems with sudden position changes.
- Cognitive symptoms ("brain fog") may impact attention, processing speed, word finding, and short-term memory — particularly affecting note taking and test taking.
- Exercise intolerance affects participation in physical activities
- Temperature sensitivity can affect comfort and concentration.
- Symptoms often fluctuate throughout the day and from day to day.

While these impacts can be significant, they can usually be effectively managed with appropriate accommodations. Based on experience with other students with this condition, the following accommodations have often proved helpful:

Physical Considerations:

- Ability to sit instead of stand during lengthy activities.
- Permission to keep prescribed medications available and take as scheduled.
- Access to water and salt-containing snacks.
- Permission to wear compression garments.
- Access to temperature-controlled environments.
- Use of elevators where available.
- Ability to leave class briefly if needed.
- Seating near doors for easy exits.
- Scheduling classes with rest periods between them.
- Choice of classroom locations to minimise walking distances.
- Access to quiet spaces for rest during breaks.
- Private changing areas for compression garments.
- Assistance with compression garments if needed.

Academic Considerations:

- Permission for water and salt during tests.
- Extended time for tests and assignments.
- Scheduling tests for optimal symptom times (often mornings).
- Flexible attendance during symptom flares.
- Permission for breaks during exams.
- Access to class notes when absent.
- Permission to record lectures.
- Use of laptop/tablet for notes if writing is fatiguing.
- Ability to complete work at home during flares.
- Alternative assignment formats when needed.
- Options for online/hybrid learning.
- Flexibility with group project participation.
- Support in planning for field trips and special events.

Physical Activity Considerations:

- Modified activities based on exercise physiologist recommendations.
- Alternative options during symptom flares.

- Flexibility to adjust participation based on daily symptoms.
- Permission to sit out when necessary.
- Option for lighter activities.
- Ready access to water and rest areas.

Special Event Planning:

- Advance planning for field trips.
- Considerations for formal events and graduations.
- Modified participation in sports days.
- Arrangements for other special occasions.

[Student Name] is managing their condition with appropriate medical care and is motivated to succeed in their studies. The specifics of which accommodations would be most helpful and feasible in your educational setting can be discussed directly with [Student Name] and their family.

Please contact me if you require any additional medical information about the condition or its impacts.

Yours sincerely,

[Doctor's Name] [Qualifications]
[Contact Information]

Work:

[Date]

RE: Workplace Considerations for [Employee Name] DOB: [Date of Birth]

To Whom It May Concern:

I am writing regarding my patient, [Name], who has Postural Orthostatic Tachycardia Syndrome (POTS), a form of Dysautonomia. This medical condition affects the autonomic nervous system, which controls involuntary body functions including heart rate, blood pressure, and temperature regulation.

Medical Impact on Work Activities: [Name]'s condition causes symptoms that can affect their workplace participation in the following ways:

- Physical symptoms including dizziness and fatigue can make prolonged standing difficult.
- Blood pressure regulation issues can cause problems with sudden position changes.
- Cognitive symptoms ("brain fog") may impact attention and processing speed.
- Exercise intolerance affects mobility around the workplace.
- Temperature sensitivity can affect comfort and concentration.
- Symptoms often fluctuate throughout the day and from day to day.

These symptoms can be effectively managed with appropriate workplace arrangements. Based on experience with other employees with this condition, the following accommodations have often proved helpful:

Physical Workspace Considerations:

- Ability to work primarily from a seated position.
- Ready access to water and salt-containing snacks.

- Permission to wear compression garments.
- Workstation located to minimise walking distances.
- Access to temperature-controlled environments.
- Use of elevators where available.
- Access to quiet rest areas when needed.
- Seating near amenities/exits.
- Permission to keep prescribed medications at desk.
- Ergonomic assessment of workstation setup.

Work Schedule Considerations:

- Flexible start times if morning symptoms are severe.
- Regular breaks for movement and position changes.
- Option for remote work during symptom flares.
- Adjusted hours to avoid peak commute times if needed.
- Time allowance for medical appointments.
- Gradual return to work after illness or leave.

Meeting and Travel Considerations:

- Option to sit during lengthy meetings.
- Permission to stand/move during traditionally seated activities.
- Ability to step out briefly if needed.
- Access to online meeting options when appropriate.
- Modified business travel arrangements if required.
- Support for off-site work requirements.

Additional Support Measures:

- Clear communication channels for difficult days.
- Flexibility with work location (office/remote).
- Understanding of day-to-day symptom variation.
- Modified emergency evacuation procedures if needed.
- Parking close to building entrance if possible.
- Support in planning for special workplace events.

Optional Section:

Graduated Return to Work Plan: Based on [Name]'s current medical status, a graduated return to work program is recommended. The following structure has proven successful for others with this condition, though the specific schedule should be adjusted based on individual response:

Week 1–2:

- 2–3 half days per week, spaced apart (e.g. Monday/Thursday).
- Focus on core tasks only.
- Preferably morning shifts when symptoms are typically better managed.

Weeks 3–4:

- 3–4 half days per week.
- Gradual introduction of additional responsibilities.
- Mix of morning and afternoon shifts to assess optimal timing.

Weeks 5–6:

- 4–5 half days or 2–3 full days.
- Increasing task complexity.
- Continue identifying optimal work patterns.

Weeks 7–8:

- Building to full days as tolerated.
- Integration of all work responsibilities.
- Establishment of sustainable work patterns.

Key Principles:

- Progress should be <u>based on symptom response rather than fixed timeframes</u>.

- Flexibility to adjust the schedule based on day-to-day variation.
- Regular review and adjustment of the plan as needed.
- Option to maintain some work-from-home days if beneficial.
- Clear communication channels to discuss any challenges.

[Name] is managing their condition with appropriate medical care and is committed to being a productive employee. The specifics of which accommodations would be most helpful and feasible in your workplace setting can be discussed directly with [Name].

Please contact me if you require any additional medical information about the condition or its impacts.

Yours sincerely,

[Doctor's Name] [Qualifications]
[Contact Information]

Travel:

[Date]

RE: Travel Considerations for [Passenger Name] DOB: [Date of Birth]

To Whom It May Concern:

I am writing regarding my patient, [Name], who has Postural Orthostatic Tachycardia Syndrome (POTS), a form of Dysautonomia. This medical condition affects the autonomic nervous system, which controls involuntary body functions including heart rate, blood pressure, and temperature regulation.

Medical Impact During Travel: [Name]'s condition causes symptoms that can be particularly challenging during travel:

- Blood pressure regulation issues can cause dizziness or fainting with prolonged standing.
- Blood pooling in legs during immobility can worsen symptoms.
- Temperature sensitivity can affect comfort and wellbeing.
- Physical fatigue can make covering long distances difficult.
- Symptoms often worsen with dehydration or heat.
- Effects can be exacerbated by travel stress and disrupted routines.

Medical Necessities During Travel: Based on managing these impacts, the following items are medically necessary:

- Prescribed medications: [list medications]
- Compression garments (must be worn during travel).
- Salt tablets and electrolyte drinks.
- Adequate water supplies exceeding standard carry-on liquid restrictions.
- Small salty snacks for symptom management.
- Any prescribed mobility aids.

Recommended Travel Accommodations: Experience with other patients suggests the following arrangements can help:

Airport/Station Assistance:

- Wheelchair assistance in terminals to minimise prolonged standing.
- Priority check-in/boarding to avoid prolonged queuing.
- Assistance with luggage when needed.
- Use of elevators or escalators rather than stairs.
- Access to seating in queuing areas if available.

During Transport:

- Seating with extra legroom when possible.
- Aisle seat for easier movement.
- Easy access to toilets.
- Permission to stand/walk periodically.
- Understanding if frequent toilet visits needed.
- Temperature control if possible.

Security Considerations:

- May need to maintain compression garments during screening.
- Medical liquids exceeding standard limits.
- Medications in both carry-on and checked luggage.
- Medical devices if applicable.

[Name] understands the need to:

- Arrive early to allow time for assistance.
- Carry supporting medical documentation.
- Declare medical items at security.
- Follow all standard safety procedures.

These accommodations will help ensure safe and comfortable travel. The specific supports needed may vary depending on the journey length and type of transport.

Please contact me if you require any additional medical information about the condition or its impacts.

Yours sincerely,

[Doctor's Name] [Qualifications]
[Contact Information]

Sport and Exercise:

[Date]

RE: Exercise Facility Considerations for [Name] DOB: [Date of Birth]

To Whom It May Concern:

I am writing regarding my patient, [Name], who has Postural Orthostatic Tachycardia Syndrome (POTS), a form of Dysautonomia. This medical condition affects the autonomic nervous system, which controls involuntary body functions including heart rate, blood pressure, and temperature regulation.

Medical Impact on Exercise: [Name]'s condition affects their exercise capacity in the following ways:

- Blood pressure regulation issues can cause dizziness particularly with sudden position changes.
- Exercise tolerance must be built very gradually to avoid setbacks.
- Recovery times may be longer than typical.
- Temperature regulation can be impaired.
- Symptoms can vary significantly day to day.
- Standing still can be more problematic than moving.

While exercise is an important part of managing this condition, it needs to be conducted appropriately. Based on experience with other patients, the following considerations have proven helpful:

Equipment Access Needs:

- Priority access to recumbent exercise equipment.
- Use of seated or reclined equipment rather than upright.
- Access to equipment in less heated areas where possible.
- Permission to use equipment for longer warm-up/cool-down periods.
- Access to fans or temperature control if available.

Safety Considerations:

- Permission to exercise at lower intensities than standard programs.
- Understanding that heart rate responses may be atypical.
- Need for longer rest periods between exercises.
- Access to floor mats for horizontal exercises.
- Ready access to water and electrolyte drinks.
- Permission to keep salt-containing snacks nearby.
- Authorisation to keep prescribed medications available.

Program Modifications:

- Focus on recumbent or horizontal exercises initially.
- Gradual progression to more upright activities.
- Modified class participation if attending group sessions.
- Flexibility to adjust intensity based on daily symptoms.
- Understanding that progress may be slower than typical.
- Need to avoid prolonged standing during instruction.

Facility Access:

- Use of elevators or ramps where available.
- Access to cooler areas for exercise.
- Permission to bring support person if needed.
- Access to seated rest areas.
- Proximity to water fountains/bathrooms.
- Private changing area if needed.

Optional Swimming Facility Section:

Swimming and water-based exercise can be particularly beneficial for this condition as it:

- Provides natural compression from the water.
- Allows exercise in a horizontal position.
- Assists with temperature regulation.
- Reduces orthostatic stress.

However, specific considerations for pool use include:

Safety Needs:

- Access to pool steps/ramp rather than ladder entry/exit.
- Permission to use pool noodles or flotation aids.
- Understanding that heart rate responses may be atypical in water.
- Clear protocol for alerting lifeguards if assistance needed.
- Access to seating at pool edge for rest periods.
- Permission for support person if needed.

Facility Considerations:

- Access to warmer water where available (but not hot pools initially).
- Use of less crowded lanes/times if possible.
- Permission to do modified versions of class activities.
- Ready access to poolside hydration.
- Access to private changing areas.
- Permission to wear compression garments under swimwear if needed.
- Understanding that exit from pool may need to be gradual.

[Name] is working with an Exercise Physiologist to develop appropriate exercise protocols. The specifics of how these considerations can be implemented in your facility can be discussed directly with [Name].

Please contact me if you require any additional medical information about the condition or its impacts.

Yours sincerely,

[Doctor's Name] [Qualifications]
[Contact Information]

Insurance/Disability Documentation:

[Date]

RE: Medical Documentation for [Name] DOB: [Date of Birth]

To Whom It May Concern:

I am writing regarding my patient, [Name], whom I have been treating for Postural Orthostatic Tachycardia Syndrome (POTS), a form of Dysautonomia, since [date]. This condition affects the autonomic nervous system, which controls involuntary body functions including heart rate, blood pressure, and temperature regulation.

They also suffer from other co-morbid conditions including: [list other conditions].

These conditions frequently interact and compound each other's effects, potentially resulting in greater functional impact than might be expected from each condition individually.

Diagnosis and Testing:

- Diagnosis confirmed through [specific criteria met/tests performed — e.g. my suggested "Dynamic Standing Test"].
- Consistent pattern of postural tachycardia demonstrated by [specific findings].
- Other causes excluded through [relevant tests/specialist reviews].

Medical Symptoms: The condition manifests with the following symptoms:

- Significant increase in heart rate upon standing (specifically [numbers] if measured).
- Blood pressure dysregulation.
- Fatigue.
- Exercise intolerance.
- Cognitive difficulties ("brain fog").

- Temperature regulation issues.
- Gastrointestinal dysfunction.

Treatment Status: Current treatments include:

- [List medications and doses]
- Structured exercise program.
- Compression garments.
- Salt and fluid protocols.

[Name] has demonstrated [good/variable/etc.] compliance with treatment recommendations and has trialled the following additional interventions:

- [List previous medication trials and outcomes].
- [List other treatment approaches attempted].

While I can document the medical aspects of this condition, I recommend a formal Occupational Therapy assessment to provide detailed information about functional impacts on daily activities, as they are better placed to assess these aspects.

From a medical perspective, I observe the following impacts during clinic visits:

- [Observable impacts during appointments].
- [Measured physiological changes].
- [Any objective findings].

Regarding prognosis:

- This condition typically improves with time and appropriate treatment.
- Recovery timeframes vary significantly between individuals.
- Current evidence suggests [any relevant prognostic factors].
- Ongoing monitoring and treatment adjustment will be required.

164

Treatment Optimisation:

- Current treatments are [still being optimised/optimised but with partial response/etc].
- Additional treatments being considered include [list if applicable].
- Response to treatment has been [description].
- Compliance with recommended treatments has been [description].

Limitations in Assessment: I should note that:

- Symptoms can vary significantly day to day.
- Impact on daily activities may differ from presentation during clinic visits.
- Functional limitations are best assessed by an Occupational Therapist assessment.
- Prognosis remains uncertain and individualised.

This condition is being actively managed with ongoing monitoring and treatment adjustment as needed. While improvement is expected over time, the timeline for recovery cannot be precisely predicted and can be in the range to several years to decades.

Please contact me if you require any additional medical information about the condition or its documented impacts.

Yours sincerely,

[Doctor's Name] [Qualifications]
[Contact Information]

Housing/Accommodation:

[Date]

RE: Housing Considerations for [Name] DOB: [Date of Birth]

To Whom It May Concern:

I am writing regarding my patient, [Name], whom I have been treating for Postural Orthostatic Tachycardia Syndrome (POTS), a form of Dysautonomia, since [date]. This condition affects the autonomic nervous system, which controls involuntary body functions including heart rate, blood pressure, and temperature regulation.

They also suffer from other co-morbid conditions including: [list other conditions].

These conditions can interact and compound each other's effects, potentially resulting in greater functional impact than might be expected from each condition individually.

Medical Impact on Housing Needs: The following aspects of [Name]'s condition are relevant to housing requirements:

- Significant difficulties with prolonged standing or stairs.
- Temperature regulation problems affecting tolerance to heat.
- Blood pressure regulation issues affecting mobility.
- Fatigue impacting ability to cover long distances.
- Symptoms that can vary significantly day to day.
- Need for regular rest periods.

Based on medical necessity, the following housing features would help manage these impacts:

Essential Considerations:

- Ground floor accommodation or reliable elevator access.
- Temperature control (air conditioning) in sleeping areas.

166

- Bathroom access without navigating stairs.
- Parking or drop-off point close to entrance.
- Accessible entrance without multiple steps.

Beneficial Features:

- Location near to essential services/campus facilities.
- Shower rather than bath access (easier entry/exit).
  - Ability to sit while showering (shower chair or built-in seating).
- Space for medical equipment if needed.
- Adequate ventilation.
- Temperature control in main living areas and bedroom.

While I can document the medical basis for these needs, the specific impact on daily activities may be better assessed by an occupational therapist. The implementation and feasibility of these accommodations would need to be discussed directly with [Name].

Please contact me if you require any additional medical information about the condition or its impacts.

Yours sincerely,

[Doctor's Name] [Qualifications]
[Contact Information]

Emergency Medical Information:

Living with dysautonomia can bring unexpected challenges, especially in situations where symptoms require urgent medical attention or accommodation. This can be particularly useful when:

- Visiting an unfamiliar Emergency Department.
- Needing to quickly communicate medical needs to emergency services personnel.
- Requiring urgent treatment while away from your usual healthcare providers.
- Experiencing symptoms in public spaces where accommodations may be needed.

Setting Up Emergency Access:

- iPhone:
    - Set up Medical ID in Health app:
        - Open Health app > Your profile > Medical ID.
        - Enable "Show when Locked".
    - Add emergency contacts, conditions, medications, and allergies.
- Android (varies by phone model):
    - Look for "Emergency Information" in Settings.
    - Common paths include:
        - Settings > Safety & Emergency.
        - Settings > About Phone > Emergency Information.
        - Settings > Lock Screen > Contact Information.
    - If you can't find it, search Settings for "Emergency" or "Medical".
- Everyone:
    - Initial Setup:
        - Test that information is accessible when phone is locked.
        - Show family/friends how to access in emergency.

- Set text size large enough to be readable when stressed/unwell.
  - ○ Access and Sharing:
    - Keep a screenshot in an easily accessible photo album/gallery.
    - Share with family/travel companions.
    - Print a copy if needed for specific situations.
  - ○ Travel Considerations:
    - Consider having a translated version if traveling internationally.
  - ○ Privacy:
    - Consider what medical information you're comfortable having accessible from locked screen.

Tips for Maintenance:

- Regular Updates:
  - ○ Update medication changes promptly.
  - ○ Keep emergency contacts current.
- Security:
  - ○ Keep a secure backup in encrypted cloud storage.
  - ○ Note date of last update.
- Healthcare:
  - ○ Share with new healthcare providers.
  - ○ Update after significant medical changes.

Printing and Physical Documentation:

Similarly, having a printed card or document can be invaluable in emergency situations. While organizations like Dysautonomia International (dysautonomiainternational.org) offer wallet cards, their limited size means they can only include basic information. For more comprehensive coverage, consider:

- Creating both a concise card-sized summary for your wallet and a more detailed document for medical situations (below),

- Making multiple copies to store in different locations (wallet, phone case, car, work),
- Laminating copies for durability, and
- Sharing copies with family members and travel companions.

While pre-made cards are helpful, having documentation that's specific to your situation and ideally signed by your treating doctor can be particularly valuable when seeking emergency care away from your usual healthcare providers. This can help expedite appropriate treatment and avoid misunderstandings about your condition.

Critical Medical Alert.

Name: [Patient Name]
DOB: [Date of Birth]
Condition: Postural Orthostatic Tachycardia Syndrome (POTS)

Immediate Needs:

- May require urgent sitting/lying down.
- Blood pressure/heart rate can be irregular.
- May need immediate fluid/salt.

Emergency Treatment:

- **First Line Therapy**:
  - 2–3L Normal Saline IV over 2–3 hours.
    - This is a proven rescue therapy for this condition.
  - If IV unavailable: oral fluids and salt.

Emergency Contacts:

- [Name] [Phone]

- Backup: [Name] [Phone]
- Doctor: Dr [Name] [Phone]

Medical Details:

- Other Conditions: [List]
- Current Medications: [Key medications and doses]
- Allergies: [List]
- Additional Instructions:
    - Avoid sudden position changes.
    - Temperature regulation may be impaired.
    - [Other key points]

Healthcare Information:

- Medicare Number: [Number]
- Insurance: [Company] [Number]

Glossary

Acetylcholine: A neurotransmitter in the nervous system that plays a key role in autonomic function.

Adrenaline/Noradrenaline: Important chemical messengers in the body (also called epinephrine and norepinephrine in North America). Both are produced by the adrenal glands and (more importantly in POTS) nerve endings:

- Adrenaline (epinephrine) is often called the "fight or flight" hormone. It increases heart rate, raises blood pressure, and diverts blood to muscles for quick action.
- Noradrenaline (norepinephrine) has similar but more subtle effects, particularly on blood pressure and blood vessel tone. It's <u>especially important in maintaining blood pressure when standing up</u>.

Both play key roles in Dysautonomia, particularly in the hyperadrenergic variant where the body may be oversensitive to their effects or producing too much of them. This is why some medications used in treating Dysautonomia work by blocking or reducing their effects.

Note: The different names (adrenaline/epinephrine and noradrenaline/norepinephrine) mean exactly the same things — they're just different naming conventions used in different parts of the world.

Albumin: The most common protein in blood plasma, critical in maintaining proper blood volume and pressure.

Alpha$_1$-adrenergic agonist: A type of medication that stimulates alpha$_1$ receptors, often used to increase blood pressure.

Anaphylaxis: A severe, potentially life-threatening allergic reaction that can occur within seconds or minutes of exposure to something you're allergic to. It causes your immune system to release a flood of chemicals that can send you into shock, with symptoms including a drop in blood pressure, difficulty breathing, and loss of consciousness.

Aseptic Meningitis: Inflammation of the protective membranes covering the brain and spinal cord, not caused by bacterial infection. Can rarely occur as a side effect of certain treatments, particularly IVIG, causing severe headaches.

Atopy: A genetic tendency to develop allergic responses including hay fever, asthma, and eczema. People with atopy typically react more readily to environmental allergens than the general population.

Attention-Deficit/Hyperactivity Disorder (ADHD): A neurodevelopmental disorder characterised by persistent patterns of inattention, hyperactivity, and impulsivity that interfere with functioning or development. Studies suggest a higher prevalence of ADHD among individuals with Dysautonomia, particularly POTS, than in the general population.

Autoimmune: Relating to a condition in which the body's immune system attacks its own tissues.

Autonomic Nervous System (ANS): The part of the nervous system that controls involuntary body functions such as heart rate, blood pressure, digestion, and temperature regulation.

Beta-blocker: A class of medications that block the effects of adrenaline and similar hormones, often used to treat high blood pressure and rapid heart rate.

Biomarker: A measurable indicator of the severity or presence of some disease state.

Bradycardia: Abnormally slow heart rate, typically defined as below 60 beats per minute in adults.

Brain Cell Plasticity (Neuroplasticity): The brain's ability to form new neural connections and reorganise existing ones, particularly in response to learning or injury.

Brain Fog: A term used to describe cognitive difficulties such as problems with concentration, memory, and clear thinking. People with brain fog often report feeling mentally "fuzzy" or "cloudy". Brain fog can vary in severity and may be exacerbated by fatigue, stress, or changes in position (e.g. standing up). While not a medical term, it's widely recognised by patients and healthcare providers as a significant factor affecting daily functioning and quality of life.

Cardio-selective: A term used to describe certain medications, particularly beta-blockers, that primarily affect the heart rather than other parts of the body. Cardio-selective drugs target specific receptors in the heart, reducing their effects on other organs such as the lungs. In the context of Dysautonomia treatment, cardio-selective beta-blockers (like metoprolol or bisoprolol) may be preferred over non-selective ones (like propranolol) for patients who also have respiratory issues, as they are less likely to cause breathing difficulties. However, it's important to note that at higher doses, even cardio-selective medications can lose some of their selectivity.

Comorbidity: The presence of one or more additional conditions co-occurring with a primary condition.

Dysautonomia: A general term for conditions caused by problems with the autonomic nervous system.

Electrolytes: Essential minerals in your blood and body fluids that carry electrical charges, including sodium, potassium, chloride, and others. They are crucial for nerve function, muscle contraction, proper hydration, and maintaining the body's chemical balance.

Endothelial Dysfunction: A condition where the inner lining of blood vessels (endothelium) doesn't function properly, affecting blood flow regulation and vessel tone. This dysfunction has been identified in many POTS patients, though its exact role isn't clear.

Epstein-Barr Virus (EBV): A common virus belonging to the herpes virus family. It's best known as the primary cause of infectious mononucleosis, often called "mono" or "glandular fever". EBV infects most people at some point in their lives, often during adolescence or young adulthood. While many people experience mild or no symptoms, some develop fatigue, fever, sore throat, and swollen lymph nodes.

Ehlers-Danlos Syndrome (EDS): A group of inherited disorders that affect connective tissues, often associated with joint hypermobility.

Fibromyalgia: A chronic condition characterised by widespread musculoskeletal pain, often accompanied by fatigue, sleep problems, memory issues, and mood changes. The exact cause is unknown, but it's thought to involve how the brain and spinal cord process pain signals.

Functional Neurological Disorder (FND): A condition where patients experience real neurological symptoms (like tremors, weakness, or blackouts) without evidence of structural damage on standard tests. The symptoms are thought to arise from problems with how the brain processes signals rather than from physical damage. Sometimes diagnosed when symptoms don't fit typical neurological patterns or when tests appear normal.

H1 Blocker: A type of antihistamine that blocks histamine H1 receptors throughout the body. These receptors are involved in many processes including allergic responses, inflammation, and blood vessel function.

H2 Blocker: A type of medication that blocks histamine H2 receptors found in various tissues of the body. While commonly known for reducing stomach acid production, these receptors also play important roles in immune system function and inflammation.

HBOT (Hyperbaric Oxygen Therapy): A medical treatment where a person breathes 100% oxygen while inside a pressurised chamber at 2–2.4 times normal sea level atmospheric pressure. This is a specialised therapy, which must be delivered in medical-grade chambers under professional supervision.

Hyperadrenergic: A state where either the body shows an exaggerated response to normal levels of adrenaline-like hormones, or the nervous system releases too much of these hormones from nerve endings. This is different from conditions where the adrenal glands themselves produce excess adrenaline.

Hypermobility: Joints that stretch further than normal.

Hypovolemia: A decreased volume of circulating blood in the body.

Implementation Gap: The delay between the development of new treatments and their widespread adoption in clinical practice. This can span years or decades due to various factors including training needs, costs, and system constraints.

IVIG (Intravenous Immunoglobulin): A treatment made from donated blood plasma containing healthy antibodies. These antibodies help regulate the immune system and reduce inflammation. Common side effects can include headache (sometimes severe), fever, and nausea.

Long COVID: Also known as Post-Acute Sequelae of SARS-CoV-2 infection (PASC), this term refers to a range of new, returning, or ongoing health problems that people experience for weeks, months, or even years after being infected with the virus that causes COVID-19.

Mast Cell Activation Syndrome (MCAS): A condition where mast cells release excessive amounts of chemical mediators, causing allergy-like symptoms.

ME/CFS (Myalgic Encephalomyelitis/Chronic Fatigue Syndrome): A complex, chronic illness characterised by severe fatigue that doesn't improve with rest, post-exertional malaise (PEM), cognitive difficulties ("brain fog"), and often pain and sleep problems. The cause is not fully understood, but it may involve immune system changes, viral infections, and genetic factors. ME/CFS shares some symptoms with Dysautonomia, particularly fatigue and cognitive issues, and the two conditions can coexist.

Mineralocorticoid: A class of steroid hormones that primarily regulate electrolyte and water balance in the body. Fludrocortisone is a synthetic mineralocorticoid. Unlike glucocorticoids (such as prednisone), which can have wide-ranging effects on metabolism and the immune system, mineralocorticoids at typical doses have a more focused effect on salt and water retention. This means that fludrocortisone, when used at standard doses for Dysautonomia, generally does not carry the same risk of side effects commonly associated with glucocorticoids, such as weight gain, osteoporosis, or immune suppression.

NASA Lean Test: A simplified test for orthostatic intolerance that can be performed in a clinical setting without specialised equipment. The patient leans their shoulders and upper back against a wall with feet placed 15 cm (6 inches) from the wall, remaining still for 10 minutes. Heart rate and blood pressure are measured when lying flat before the test, and then at set intervals while leaning. A positive test for POTS is indicated by:

- In adults age 20 or over: An increase in heart rate of 30+ beats per minute

- In teenagers age 12–19yo: An increase in heart rate of 40+ beats per minute

- Or a sustained heart rate of 120+ beats per minute during the test

For orthostatic hypotension, a drop in blood pressure of more than 20/10 mmHg is considered significant.

Off-label: The use of a medication in a way that differs from its official government approval. This includes using medications for different conditions, doses, or patient groups than officially specified. While legal and common, especially for rare conditions where formal approval hasn't been sought, off-label use requires careful consideration by prescribing doctors to ensure it is supported by evidence and in the patient's best interest.

Orthostatic Hypotension: A form of low blood pressure that occurs when standing up from a sitting or lying position.

Orthostatic Intolerance: The development of symptoms when standing upright that are relieved when reclining.

Osmolar Load (Osmolality): A measure of how concentrated dissolved substances (like salts and sugars) are in food or drinks. Both the concentration and the amount matter — a larger meal will have a greater impact than a smaller one of the same concentration. In Dysautonomia, meals with a high osmolar load draw water from the blood into the digestive tract for processing, which can temporarily worsen symptoms like dizziness and fatigue.

Pacemaker: The heart's natural "timer" that controls its rhythm and rate. Located in the upper right chamber of the heart, it sends out electrical signals telling the heart when to beat. In some types of Dysautonomia, this natural pacemaker can work too fast, especially when standing up. Certain medications used to treat Dysautonomia work by helping to regulate this.

Palpitations: Medically, being aware of the sensation of your heart beating. Often with the connotation of it being unusually hard, fast, or irregular.

Parasympathetic Nervous System: A division of the autonomic nervous system that promotes "rest and digest" functions. It generally works to conserve energy and regulate bodily functions during states of calm, including slowing heart rate, increasing digestive activities, and promoting relaxation.

Parkinsonism: A group of neurological disorders that cause movement problems similar to those seen in Parkinson's disease, including tremors, slow movement, stiffness, and problems with walking and balance. It is often associated with autonomic dysfunction.

Photobiomodulation: A scientific-sounding term for light therapy, where specific wavelengths of light are applied to the body. While there is some evidence for effects on surface tissues like skin, superficial muscles or via the eyes, claims about deeper effects (particularly through the skull to the brain) are not well supported by current research. The term is often used in marketing materials to make simple light exposure sound more technologically advanced. While generally safe when proper eye protection is used, be wary of expensive devices or treatments making extravagant claims about its benefits.

Post-COVID-19 Vaccination Syndrome (PCVS): Sometimes referred to as "Long Vax", this term describes a set of symptoms that some individuals report experiencing following COVID-19 vaccination. These symptoms can be similar to those seen in Long COVID, including fatigue, brain fog, and Dysautonomia-like symptoms. It's important to note that this condition is rare, and the benefits of vaccination in preventing severe COVID-19 (and Long Covid) vastly outweigh the risks.

Post-Exertional Malaise (PEM) / "Crashes": A severe worsening of symptoms following minimal physical, cognitive, or emotional exertion. PEM typically has a delayed onset (12–48 hours post-exertion) and can last for days or weeks. Symptoms may include extreme fatigue, cognitive difficulties, muscle pain, and flu-like symptoms.

Postural Orthostatic Tachycardia Syndrome (POTS): A form of Dysautonomia characterised by an abnormal increase in heart rate upon standing.

Pre-syncope: The sensation of feeling faint or lightheaded without actually fainting.

Recumbent: A position where the body is lying down, reclining, or leaning back.

Rescue Therapy: Treatments kept in reserve for managing severe symptom flares or special circumstances, rather than for regular use. In this setting, examples might include IV saline or stellate ganglion blocks.

SNRI (Serotonin Noradrenaline Reuptake Inhibitor): A class of antidepressant medications that work by increasing the amounts of both serotonin and noradrenaline (chemical messengers) in the brain by preventing their reabsorption. Common examples include venlafaxine (Efexor/Effexor) and duloxetine (Cymbalta). Because SNRIs increase noradrenaline levels, which can affect heart rate and blood pressure, they may worsen symptoms in some people with Dysautonomia, though individual responses vary.

SSRI (Selective Serotonin Reuptake Inhibitor): A commonly prescribed class of antidepressant medications that work by increasing the amount of serotonin (a chemical messenger) available in the brain. SSRIs accomplish this by preventing the reabsorption (reuptake) of serotonin by nerve cells, leaving more serotonin available to improve transmission of messages between neurons. Common examples include sertraline (Zoloft), escitalopram (Lexapro), and fluoxetine (Prozac). Unlike some other antidepressants, SSRIs are generally well-tolerated by people with Dysautonomia and may often help a little.

Sympathetic Nervous System: A division of the autonomic nervous system that promotes "fight or flight" responses. It prepares the body for intense physical activity by increasing heart rate, blood pressure, and breathing rate, while also diverting blood flow to muscles and suppressing digestive activities.

Synapse/Synaptic: The tiny gap between nerve cells where chemical signals pass from one nerve to another. When something is described as "synaptic," it relates to these connection points. In Dysautonomia treatment, some medications work by affecting how long chemical messengers stay in these gaps, strengthening the signals between nerves.

Syncope: A temporary loss of consciousness, also known as fainting.

Syndrome: A set of symptoms or conditions that occur together and suggest the presence of a certain disease or an increased chance of developing the disease.

Tachycardia: Greek for fast (tachy) heart (cardia). Abnormally rapid heart rate, typically defined as above 100 beats per minute in adults.

Titration: The process of gradually adjusting the dose of a medication to determine the optimal dosage.

Tragus: The small piece of cartilage that partially covers your ear canal at the front. Important in some emerging treatments as it is supplied by the only branch of the vagus nerve that can be stimulated externally.

Vagus Nerve: The longest and most complex of the cranial nerves, playing a crucial role in the parasympathetic nervous system.

Vasoconstriction: The process of narrowing of blood vessels. Increases the pressure of the blood in them.

Vasodilation: The process of widening of blood vessels. Decreases the pressure of blood in them.

Vasovagal Syncope: A type of fainting caused by a sudden drop in heart rate and blood pressure, often triggered by stress or emotional upset.

Venous Pooling: The excessive collection of blood in veins, particularly in the legs, due to gravity and poor blood vessel tone. Often visible as purple blotchy discoloration and can contribute to symptoms when standing.

Made in the USA
Coppell, TX
09 March 2025

46864487R00105